In Praise of

"A Journey to Healing"

For most people there comes a time in their life when they seek "healing". Healing for ails that trouble them whether they be physical, emotional, mental or spiritual in nature. Where though does one go when in search for healing? What are the methods that heal and who are the healers?

Bruce Winkle addresses these questions in his book, A Journey to Healing – Laying the Foundation to Energetic Wellness. Written as a training handbook for energy practitioners, he takes on the complex subject: Energy Medicine, the foundational source for deep, whole and complete healing. He weaves together the healing wisdom of many ancient and indigenous traditions and builds the groundwork for understanding the main concepts and principles in energy medicine. Clearly written, he is able to simplify the complex and bring brevity to the lengthy. His relatively short exploration of these concepts is surprisingly comprehensive, and serves as a welcomed joy to the reader.

The main thrust of his writing focuses on training the energy practitioner. Blending ancient foundational principles of energy medicine with his own discoveries about energy and healing, Bruce brings original thought to the subject and defines a method for healing. He expands on the concept of cellular memory and cellular vibration, and how wounds from the past and trauma are held in the body. This framework and approach takes into account working on all the layers of the body and thus embraces a system of healing on all levels: mind, emotions, body and spirit.

Being an energy medicine practitioner myself, and aligning with Bruce's thoughts, I was quite impressed with how he synthesized the information and formatted the healing protocol into a step by step format that can be easily understood by the intermediate energy medicine practitioner. His style of writing is very succinct, easy to understand and is further complemented by simple, tasteful illustrations. The student is very fortunate to have this type of training manual for it serves as a clear guidebook that one can come back to time and time again. Philosophical quotes grace each chapter and create space for personal reflection and contemplation.

I applaud Bruce for having the courage and stamina to synthesis all that he has learned from his studies, experiences and guidance and to offer us all his wisdom about healing with a well-defined protocol for energy practitioners and healers. Well done!

Suzanne Nixon, EdD, LPC, LMFT, RMT
Licensed Professional Counselor
Licensed Marriage and Family Therapist
Certified Massage Therapist & Energy Medicine Practitioner

A Journey to Healing

Laying the Foundation
to Energetic Wellness

Bruce Winkle

A Journey to Healing

Laying the Foundation
to Energetic Wellness

Energy Flow

Lifelines

Chakras

Expanding
Energy Flow

Gateways
to Emotions

Energies
of the Heart

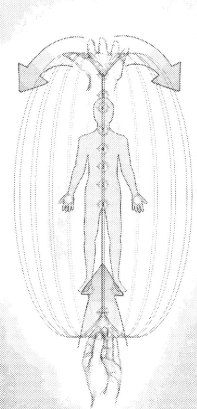

Bruce Winkle

A Journey to Healing

bruce@brucewinkle.com   www.brucewinkle.com

Illustrations by Penny Hauffe
www.pennypaints.com

Printed in the United States of America

Published by: Merrazz-LLC
Leesburg, VA 20176
www.merrazz-LLC.com

First Edition 2015

US $ 24.95

ISBN: 978-0-9846868-2-7

Disclaimer

The material in this handbook is a guide for energy healing for yourself and others. It is not a replacement for traditional health care, medical diagnosis or medical treatments including prescribed medications for illness. Please refer to a licensed medical practitioner for medical care.

A Journey to Healing

Laying the Foundation to Energetic Wellness

Contents

	Page #
Introduction	7
World of Energy	8
Energy Medicine	9
Energy in Medicine	10
Clearing Held Memories Story	11
Chapter 1	13
The Journey Begins	
Chapter 2	25
Chakras	
Chapter 3	35
Energy Flow	
Chapter 4	47
Energy Flow and Chakras	
Chapter 5	57
Expanding Energy Flow	
Chapter 6	73
Gateways to Emotion	
Chapter 7	87
Energies of the Heart	
Chapter 8	105
Lifelines	
Appendix	123
Suggested Readings	125
For All the Ladies	126
Training Program	128
Bruce's Bio	133

"Our chief want is someone

who will inspire us to be

what we know we could be."

Ralph Waldo Emerson

In Gratitude

I am grateful to my many wonderful friends, teachers, students and clients both animal and human, whom have helped me understand the special wonders of energy healing and have helped me become the healer and teacher I am today.

In addition, I wish to extend my heartfelt thanks to each of you who has and who will join with me on this special journey to healing.

Bruce Winkle

A Journey to Healing

<u>With Sincere Appreciation To</u>

Alma Zarate and Tonia Bultrowicz for their support and assistance in compiling notes and suggestions from my workshops and classes.

Donna Coleman for her dancing fingers on the computer keyboard.

Nancy & Bruce Mountz for their encouragement of my training programs.

Eileen Frumkin for her wonderful proof reading.

Samantha Macher for her editing suggestions.

Special appreciation to Penny Hauffe for her wonderful artistic illustrations that assist me in presenting this material to you. Please visit her website to learn more about this wonderful artist.   www.pennypaints.com

A very special thank you to

My wife, Claudia, for her daily encouragement and support of
my journey into this wonderful world of energy healing.
She brings sunshine into my life.

Bruce Winkle

Introduction

The objective of this handbook is to present the foundation of a unique and powerful form of energetic bodywork. This work includes energy systems and essential procedures that support the energetic health and well-being of all life.

You will be introduced to energy aspects, viewpoints, and entryways to the body's held emotions. New perceptions will expand your understanding of how our energy systems connect and flow within our bodies.

Insightful techniques will empower you with ways to clear and heal the wonderful and powerful Heart. Additional wisdom will show you how to release deeply held traumatic events that are held within in the energetic Life Line of a body.

By bringing this knowledge together you will be able to help yourself and your clients release many old injuries and limiting beliefs that may be standing in the way of profound healing.

The information and insights in this handbook are from the knowledge I have acquired by studying many diverse energy healing modalities, as well as my ongoing energy healing work with people and animals.

A World of Energy

In today's modern world, we truly live in an ocean of energy. This ocean of energetic frequencies and vibrations includes various forms of electromagnetic fields, sounds, transmissions, visible and non-visible light spectrums, and the Earth's bio-rhythms.

Hundreds of scientific studies over the last fifty years have consistently revealed that this wide spectrum of energetic frequencies and vibrations profoundly impact every facet of our biological systems.

The electromagnetic fields that permeate our bodies include those sent out by our earth, moon and sun. We are also greatly affected by microwave, ovens, TVs, computers, electrical transmission lines and many testing and/or diagnostic instruments. These disruptions or imbalances to our body's energy fields may even correlate to illness.

Sounds from traffic, blaring broadcasts, industrial plants, construction sites and many yard care items such as lawn mowers, leaf blowers, snow blowers, and household appliances also have a major effect on our nervous systems.

The vast array of satellite, television, radar, radio, wireless and cellular communications which surround us daily also and permeate us as well. The visible and non-visible light spectrums including sun burst, light fixtures and the amount of natural light we receive affect us too. All of these vibrations have a major effect on both our immune and energy systems.

Energy and Matter

As we learned in science class, atoms are the building blocks of matter and are composed of protons, neutrons, and electrons. With new technologies scientists have discovered that protons, neutrons, and electrons are not particles themselves, but are actually subtle vibrations.

The density at which vibrations combine determines the type of matter they will form - whether it is the stars, earth, trees, bone, muscle or organs.

Everything in our world is vibrations or energy in one form or another. Whether it is our thoughts, feelings, emotions or physical matter including animal, vegetable, and mineral - it is comprised of energy. Nothing is truly solid.

Energy Medicine

Modern allopathic or Western medicine has divided our bodies into many systems. These include our cardiovascular, skeletal, nervous, endocrine, immune, urinary and reproductive systems. However, we are far more than just a collection of cells and biochemical reactions.

Energy is the basis for all forms of the physical, emotional, mental and spiritual aspects of all life. It is energy that connects us to all other forms of life and is the missing essence of the modern Western medicine model.

The ancient concept of energy medicine has existed in every culture throughout history. For thousands of years, Qi or Chi has been the energetic force of health described in Oriental or Eastern Medicine. Prana has been the vital energy in Ayurveda medicine. Indigenous peoples have always viewed health in terms of life force or Spirit.

Energy Medicine, also called Vibrational Medicine, is based on the scientific principles that all matter, including the human body, is in fact pulsating energy, with each feature vibrating at a precise frequency. Today's scientists are able to identify the various compounds in a mixture, as well as far off stars in our universe, by the unique frequencies to which each form of matter vibrates.

The natural state of a healthy and balanced energy system is the ability to pulsate in and out of stillness and movement easily. In other words the ability to flow without restrictions. Traumas often result in energy states of either no movement or constant movement. Contrary to what you might think, the body wisely creates these states in order not to overwhelm itself when traumas occur.

However, when traumas are recorded deeply, the body is unable to self-correct. When the body's energy ceases to flow freely, it allows portions to become stagnate, and over time disease may set in. If parts of the body never rest, these parts will eventually burn out their natural defenses and then may also allow disease to set in.

Energy in Medicine

With new equipment developed to follow the principles of bioenergy, today's physicians are able to more accurately diagnose disease. These technologies analyze internal problems by distinguishing the energy characteristics of organs and tissues. *Healthy* tissue emits its own unique energy signature, which differs from the energy emitted by the same type of *diseased* tissue.

The use and efficiency of the diagnostic instruments that read our body's bioenergy fields is truly amazing. These instruments include: CAT, PET, MRI, EKG, EEG, EMG, MEG, Thermal Imaging and Ultrasound.

Physicians also use energy waves to break up kidney stones, and electrical wave stimulators to facilitate bone healing. TENS, ultra-sound, and cold lasers are used to release stagnation in muscles. Instruments such as pacemakers and defibrillators are also widely used in medical treatments.

Therapeutic Energy

Throughout the ages, there have always been some people who can easily feel or see energy as it flows within, around and beyond the physical body. Some instruments have even been developed to aid in perceiving this energy, commonly referred to as the "Aura," such as Kirlian and Aura photography.

With some instruction, most people can feel, sense or see this life force energy and utilize it in their own health and healing. Those who can accurately sense the energy and how it moves, can assist the rest of us by using various techniques to make healing an easy and natural process.

Responsibility for our health ultimately lies with each of us. Energy governs all life, and all life forms are inseparable from one another. By helping ourselves, we ultimately help everyone in our global community.

Now, believe that you can learn how to connect with the universal energy to which we all have access, and provide yourself a wonderful way to share healing for yourself, your loved ones and all living things.

A Journey to Healing

The *Clearing Held Memories* Story

As each of us proceeds on our personal life journey, we may encounter traumas on a physical, mental, emotional and/or spiritual level. These may include the death of a loved one, loss of a job, loss of friends, physical injuries, accidents, divorce and/or stress at work.

When these traumatic events occur, we keep moving forward by burying it deep within ourselves, perhaps thinking we will release the issue at a later time. Unfortunately, more often than not, we never go back and revisit the issue thinking we have already dealt with it.

During my early years of sharing energy work with clients, specifically those who had or who were recovering from cancer, I felt that they were not fully releasing their deeply held traumatic memories. These memories invariably held back their full return to a vibrant state of being.

With that realization, I decided to challenge myself and discover how to facilitate the release of these held traumatized cellular vibrations on both their physical and energetic levels.

While continuing to study many healing traditions as well as current medical research, I began to understand how the body and energy systems record traumas.

The one thing that continued to be evident was that each cell has its own memory and is connected to other cells which could be holding traumatized memories. Ironically, as cells die off and are replaced by new ones, those memories are transferred to the new cells. Therefore, the cycle of trapped memories held in our tissues can continue to create imbalances in the energy flow of our bodies.

By understanding that connecting to the cellular and energetic components of traumatized memories is a major key in restoring a person's vitality, I was able to develop the *Clearing Held Memories* Training Program.

The knowledge and techniques that form the foundation of this unique and powerful form of energetic bodywork are presented in this handbook.

Chapter 1

The

Journey

Begins

"We have a hunger of the mind

which asks for knowledge of all around us,

and the more we gain,

the more is our desire;

the more we see,

the more we are capable of seeing."

Maria Mitchell

The Journey Begins

Ethics Guidelines

The foundation of this unique form of energetic bodywork and the techniques used involve touching the client while the client remains clothed. The techniques may also be used directly on a client during a massage or other licensed touch therapy session.

If you are new to energetic bodywork and have not taken a Bodyworkers Ethics course please review and follow the guidelines below when using these techniques with your family, friends and future clients.

1. If you are not a licensed massage, medical or religious therapist, please check your local licensing board to confirm touch is allowed under your therapy license.

2. Safeguard the confidentiality of all client information, unless disclosure is requested by the client in writing, is medically necessary, is required by law, or necessary for the protection of the public.

3. Respect the client's right to treatment with informed and voluntary consent. Obtain informed consent of the client, or client's advocate, prior to providing treatment. This consent may be written or verbal.

4. Respect the client's right to refuse, modify or terminate treatment regardless of prior consent given.

5. Provide treatment in a way that ensures the safety, comfort and privacy of the client.

6. Respect the client's boundaries with regard to privacy, disclosure, exposure, emotional expression, beliefs and the client's reasonable expectations of professional behavior.

7. Follow the National Certification Board for Therapeutic Massage and Bodywork Standards of Practice, Code of Ethics, and all policies, procedures and guidelines.

8. Follow all regulations, codes, and requirements of your state and local licensing boards.

The Journey Begins

Becoming an Energy Practitioner

Heal Thyself First

The number one goal healers should incorporate into their daily lives is self-care. As healers, we get caught up in our desire to help others. We begin to think that as energy healers we do not need self-care because we get the overflow or extra energy that we are helping channel to our clients. However, to be the best and clearest channel for healing energy we need to include self-care into every day.

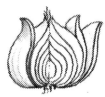 Just like an onion, we have many layers that have accumulated during our journeys'. Our goal is to keep peeling away the layers of past traumatic events to become the best healing vessel we can be!

Take the time to receive energy and/or bodywork.

Work on yourself each day.

Be the clearest channel you can be.

Self-Care

In addition to learning new knowledge and experiencing new techniques while reading this handbook you will also be experiencing self-healing. This self-healing may be on a much deeper level than you have experienced before.

To be sure that your body is not overwhelmed with the deep releases of toxins and emotions, it is highly recommended that you begin a daily routine of self-care.

The following suggestions will not only help your body release toxins, but will also increase the flow of energy throughout your entire system. This new found energy will not only help you in your personal life, but will also help deepen your connection to this wonderful new work you will be learning.

<u>Suggestions</u>

<u>Self-Talk</u> - Make time to have positive talks with <u>yourself</u>.

> What is your daily self-talk like?
>
> Are you positive about <u>you</u>?
>
> Do you scold or beat yourself up?
>
> Do you remind yourself you are a child of the divine?

<u>Living Environment Changes</u>

Make changes to your living environment to support your changing vibration to a higher level.

Look at your surroundings and make changes that bring you a calmer outlook on your life. (Color, artwork, furniture layout, and even clutter.)

What type of background music (sounds) do you listen to? Does it support calmness or is it the negative news?

<u>Diet Changes</u>

There are many good books and dietary practitioners that can guide you to what is right for you.

One of the easiest ways to start is to review of your current diet.
Whenever possible, eliminate fast food, added salt, sugars and stimulants

Add a high quality <u>probiotic</u> to your daily supplement program, available at your local health food store or the health department of a holistic food store.

To receive the highest benefit from the probiotic purchase one that has been refrigerated since production and that you continue to keep refrigerated. This maintains the potency which may be reduced if stored at higher temperatures.

The Journey Begins

Self-Care Suggestions Continued

Sound Meditation

Listen to chakra meditation music every day at least one chakra per day.

CD recommendations

Chakra Chants by Jonathan Goldman
Chakra Chants 2 by Jonathan Goldman
Music for Sound Healing by Steven Halpern
Spectrum Suite by Steven Halpern

Epson Salt Footbaths

Obtain a plastic tub that is a minimum of 12" wide x 17" long and 7" deep. Place ½ cup of Epson Salts in as hot of water as your feet can stand without scalding.

Soak your feet for 20 to 25 minutes while you insulate your body with sweat pants and hooded sweatshirt or wrapped in towels.

The intention is to create an individual sweat lodge to increase circulation of blood and the lymph system.

Small & Large Intestinal Cleanse

Begin taking natural Psyllium Husks which can be found at your local health food stores.

Directions: Start with one level teaspoon in 4-6 ounces of water, in the evening for one week. Then on week two, increase to one rounded teaspoon morning and evening. Week three increase the evening dose to one tablespoon. Week four will increase to one rounded tablespoon in the morning.
Maintain the rounded tablespoon morning and evening for a minimum of three months.

Law of the Cure

Like many other healing modalities, the techniques you will learn in this handbook assists the body in healing itself.

During the healing process, a pattern emerges which has been documented by homeopaths, acupuncturists, chiropractors, and even psychologists. This pattern is referred to as the Law of the Cure.

This Law indicates that in natural healing, symptoms from past physical, mental or emotional traumas often briefly reoccur in order to clear.

As with deep massage sessions, there is always the possibility that you may feel worse before you feel better after an energy healing session. This is especially true when the session helped clear some deeply held issues.

It is important to remember that you should plan a day or so for yourself to allow your body to process these clearings. It is recommended that you not schedule a session a couple of days before an important event.

You may also experience some of the following symptoms during the 24 to 48 hours following a session.

> Lethargy
> Stand-offish-ness
> Irritability
> Soreness or aching areas on your body
> Mood swings, and/or not knowing where emotions are coming from
> Feeling like you want to stay in bed and pull the covers over your head
> Having dark urine with possible stronger odors than normal
> Loose stools
> A low fever
> Bloated or gassy

Allow yourself to process and release the issues that have been brought up by the session. Keep an eye on the symptoms that arise, but as much as possible allow the clearing to take place.

Try not to take medication to reduce what is commonly referred to as the toxicity release.

Practitioner Preparation

Prior to Conducting a Healing Session

Know your boundaries, and when it's not the time to practice.

Get a good night sleep before you facilitate a healing session.

Be sure you are fully grounded.

Center and focus yourself before you connect.

Make sure you stay hydrated.

Your Healing Space

Make sure your chair and table are at the right height for you. Hands should be at the level of the client's feet.

Have a blanket/or sheet available for the client's comfort.

Have your props within reach to ensure you don't get fatigued.

Props: arm support pillow or rolled up sheet. Also you may use the

table or your client's body (if necessary) as a prop within reason.

Have a clock within sight and your music selected.

Remember to always treat a person's energy with respect. When connecting, disconnecting or moving between connection points, do so gently – not suddenly or abruptly, and with gentle intention.

Your Client

Ask permission to touch, and acknowledge any reservations they may have. If necessary, review some of the hand placements.

Make sure their heels are on the table and not hanging over the edge, as this can cut the energy off.

Place a pillow or bolster under their knees to support their low back.

Session Notes

Reconfirm your client is comfortable.

When you cover your client with a sheet or blanket, you will then need to uncover, or roll back, the area you will be working on. This is known as draping. Do not reach under the covering.

Keys to Energy Healing

Focus ….What are you working on? Let the energy know.

Intention….What do you want to do with what you are working on?

As an energy practitioner, you are here to be a conduit for healing. Do not set or expect certain results, but **allow** the healing that is correct for your client at this time to take place. This does not mean to be uninvolved, but to allow what is right for the client to happen with no judgment.

Breathe! Remember to breathe in a rhythmic manner. A rhythmic pattern ensures that all the carbon dioxide produced by the body will be eliminated and that enough oxygen will come into the body. This will also facilitate your centering and grounding.

There are clients that may see colors when they are connected during sessions. It is not as much about what color, but the density or thickness of the color. The more translucent the colors, the higher and clearer the vibration.

Ways to recognize changes in the energy

As you are working with you own or another person's energy be aware of the subtle changes that occur in the energy. Changes such as:

Smoothness	Thickness
Coldness	Heat
Pulsation	Lack of spikes
Jumpiness	Erratic pulse
Very quiet	Shift in vibration

The Journey Begins

Session Notes Continued

Paying attention to the non-verbal behavior of your clients will give you feedback on how the session is shifting your client's energy.

Possible responses when energy imbalances are being released

Body relaxing	Allowing the mouth to relax
Fluttering/or twitching	Jerking movements
Nausea	Chills
Burping or gas	Feeling ill
Pain	Yawning or snoring
Tingling	Laughing
Tears	Crying out loud

As a new energy healer you may also experience clients that release lots of verbal emotions. If this happens pause the session but stay connected. If the verbal release continues for some time go to the feet and ground your client for as long as it takes to allow them to work through their release.

Do not engage in any verbal response even though you may feel drawn to do so. Remember you are there to support their process and are not a counselor.

 Remember, just like layers of an onion, we are helping peel off accumulations of old events held within the cells of the body.

If you feel stagnation attached to you at the end of a session, take time to re-ground yourself and allow the stagnation to flow to the earth.

NOTE: Animals have the same energy systems as humans. Use the same focus and intention when sharing energy work with them.

<u>Healing Notes</u>

"If change didn't happen, there would be no butterflies."

1 - As an energy worker, you are now creating a dialog or conversation between you and the energy. Be sure you use the same focus and clarity of intentions each time you connect so you will get the response you are asking for. Don't change the language of the conversation each time you connect.

2 - Clear what needs to be cleared for the energy to shift, and don't get caught up in the drama of any particular event that may have facilitated the shift.

3 - Help those you are treating to take responsibility for their own healing so that they may hold their true power. This means that our first concern, and our first intent, must always be to find ways to facilitate others' healing without taking power from them.

4 - A person's vibration and energy will respond despite any formal ability by you to send healing. So be sure you are holding the highest intent for each session.

5 - Be sure to ground <u>yourself</u> before releasing from your client. You can do this by holding both ankles of your client, set your intention and use energy flow to ground your chakras with the Earth.

6 - When a person comes in scattered and very talkative, consider connecting to the head to ground the scattered energy. Keep in mind you are still moving energy up from the Earth, through the body to the head. Gently return the energy down the outside of the body to the Earth. Repeat until the scattered energy feels grounded.

<u>Healing Notes Continued</u>

7 - Always be on the alert for any unusually quiet areas of energy. These areas are a sure sign that something is being hidden and will need to be addressed for the healing process to fully take place.

8 - Our true strength as healers lies in being able to be vulnerable. It is our humanness that makes us special. We must learn to let this shine through in all that we do, and share mistakes openly with others. In this way, our perceived weaknesses will soon become our greatest strengths.

9 - Understand that illness is not always a sign that something is wrong. There are times when illness is necessary to facilitate change, and our role is to help facilitate that process.

10 - What happens when you or your client do not feel the session made a difference?

One or both of you came with expectations for clearing a symptom. Many times, the client's primary symptom is the last item to clear after the body is in balance and has returned to harmony.

11 – You can only be responsible <u>to</u> your clients. You are not responsible <u>for</u> your clients.

12 – Become aware of the various subtleties of energy vibrations. These intricacies of energy will begin to guide you to where the clearing should take place.

Chapter 2

Chakras

"Look deep into nature,

and

you will understand everything better."

Albert Einstein

Introducing the Chakras

We begin our look at energy systems with the Chakras. Most or all of you are aware of these wonderful energy centers that are present throughout the body.

The word Chakra is of Sanskrit origin (an ancient language of India) meaning vortex or spinning wheel. These spinning energy centers are responsible for bringing in fresh energies for the body to use, and also to remove any stagnate or used energy from the body.

Chakras also imprint records, or memories, of past traumatic events (physical, mental, emotional, and/or spiritual) in a person's life. These records/memories may be recorded in more than one chakra and form restrictions to the flow of energy within the body.

Recorded memories may also restrict the release of stagnate energy out of the body. Restriction of stagnate energy makes the release of old habits and behaviors very difficult.

Each Chakra resonates at its own unique vibrational rate which is needed for the body systems it serves. They begin with a slower vibration of (approximately 256-Hz) at the Root Chakra and increase in vibrational rate up to (approximately 480-Hz) at the Crown Chakra. Each unique vibrational rate corresponds to a select color range which also vibrates at the same rate.

The unique vibration of each Chakra influences the organs, glands, muscles, veins and all systems within its energy field. This vibrational energy also influences the endocrine system (hormones) and is strongly involved with our moods, personality, and our overall health.

The core, or centers of the major body Chakras are positioned along a column of energy that parallels the inside portion of the spine. They begin at the base of the spine with the Root Chakra and proceed up the body to the Crown Chakra which is located on the top of the head.

On the illustration page that follows, you will see the Chakras and their location, as we will be referring to them in this handbook. The illustration includes the traditional seven major body Chakras as well as the Earth and the 8th Chakra.

Chakra Locations

Chakra Name		Location
Transpersonal Star	**8**	6" to several feet above the top of the head.
Crown	**7**	On the top of the head.
Brow	**6**	Just above the center of the eye brows.
Throat	**5**	At the base of the throat.
Heart	**4**	In the middle of the chest.
Solar Plexus	**3**	Slightly below the base of the sternum.
Sacral	**2**	At the top of the sacrum at the point of the hips.
Root	**1**	At the bottom of the body at the pubic area.
Earth	Earth	6" to several feet, in the ground, below the bottom of your feet.

Summary of the Chakras

8 – Transpersonal Star - Transforms higher energies into physical energy.

7 - Crown Chakra - Spirituality, Selflessness.
Governs: top center of the head and midline above the ears, brain, nervous system, pineal gland.

6 - Brow Chakra - Intuition, Wisdom.
Governs: brain, eyes, ears, nose, pituitary gland, pineal gland, neurological system.

5 - Throat Chakra - Communication, Self-expression.
Governs: throat, thyroid gland, parathyroid gland, trachea, cervical vertebrae, vocal cords, neck, shoulder, arms, hands, esophagus, mouth, teeth, gums.

4 - Heart Chakra - Love and Relationships.
Governs: heart, rib cage, blood, circulatory system, lungs and diaphragm, thymus gland, breasts, esophagus, shoulders, arms, hands.

3 - Solar Plexus - Personal power, Self-will.
Governs: upper abdomen, gallbladder, liver, middle spine, kidney, adrenals, small intestines, stomach.

2 - Sacral Chakra - Emotional balance, Belonging.
Governs: sexual organs, stomach, large intestines, liver, gallbladder, kidney, pancreas, adrenal glands, spleen, middle spine, auto immune system.

1 - Root Chakra - Physical survival and needs.
Governs: bones, teeth, nails, anus, prostate, adrenals, kidneys, lower digestive functions, excretory functions, and sexual activity.

Earth Chakra - Transforms earth energy into physical energy

Chakra Strengths

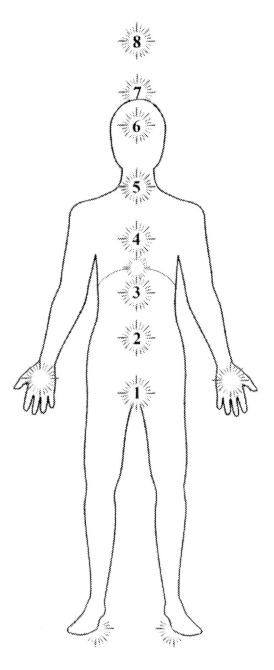

8- Strong connection to guidance from your higher self.

7- Feeling at one with the universe, open-minded, thoughtful, understand and learn information more easily.

6- Ability to think reality into existence, imagination, intuition, concentration and focus.

5- Creative and expressive, constructive communication, contentment, conscious listening, positive self-expression.

4- Feeling of completeness, compassionate, empathic, friendly, optimistic, motivated, nurturing, and outgoing.

3- Energetic, confident, intelligent, decisive, productive, good digestion, mental focus.

2- Compassionate, friendly, intuitive, vital, sexual, prosperous, satisfied, having a sense of belonging and humor.

1- Connected to your body, centered, having energy and vitality, able to digest foods well.

E- Well grounded, able to release strong emotions as they happen.

Chakras

Physical & Emotional Issues

Crown - **Physical Dysfunctions:** chronic exhaustion, sensitivity to light and sound.

    Emotional Issues: disbelief in any spiritual realities, selflessness, apathy, sense of fear, materialism. Lack of: purpose, devotion, identity, inspiration, trust, values and ethics.

Brow - **Physical Dysfunctions:** headaches, nightmares, eyestrain, depression, learning disabilities, panic, blindness, deafness, seizures, spinal dysfunctions.

    Emotional Issues: evaluation, concept of reality and confusion. Fear of truth and, discipline. Lack of concentration and judgment.

Throat - **Physical Dysfunctions:** thyroid dysfunctions, sore throat, stiff neck, mouth ulcers, swollen glands, gum or tooth problems, teeth grinding, scoliosis, laryngitis, hearing problems.

    Emotional Issues: faith, will and addiction. Fear of: decision making, personal expression, creativity and criticism.

Heart - **Physical Dysfunctions:** thoracic spine, upper back and shoulder problems, asthma, heart conditions, shallow breathing, lung disease.

    Emotional Issues: difficulty with love, despair, moody, envy, fear, jealousy, anger and anxiety. Lack of: hope, compassion and confidence.

Solar Plexus - **Physical Dysfunctions:** diabetes, pancreatitis, adrenal imbalances, arthritis, colon diseases, stomach ulcers, intestinal tumors, anorexia/bulimia, low blood pressure.

    Emotional Issues: timid, depression, inability to make decisions, judgmental, perfectionism, anger, rage, hostility. Fear of rejection. Lack of self-esteem and self-image.

Sacral - **Physical Dysfunctions:** lower back pain, sciatica, decreased libido, pelvic pain, urinary problems, poor digestion, low resistance to infection and viruses, tiredness, hormonal imbalances, menstrual problems.

    Emotional Issues: irritability, shyness, guilt, blame, sexual obsession. Lack of: power, money, control, creativity and morality.

Root - **Physical Dysfunctions:** tiredness, poor sleep, lower back pain, sciatica, constipation, depression, immune related disorders, obesity and eating disorders.

    Emotional Issues: ungrounded, afraid, rage, anger, obsessed with comfort, alienated, possessive. Lack of: self- esteem, survival and security.

Stirring the Chakras

An easy to way to clear stagnant energy located in a chakra is to use the stirring technique. To visualize the stirring technique, imagine extending the energy of your fingers into a fishbowl (which would represent a chakra). Now gently stir the energy in the selected chakra in a clockwise motion until all areas, top, right, left and the bottom feel clear and smooth.

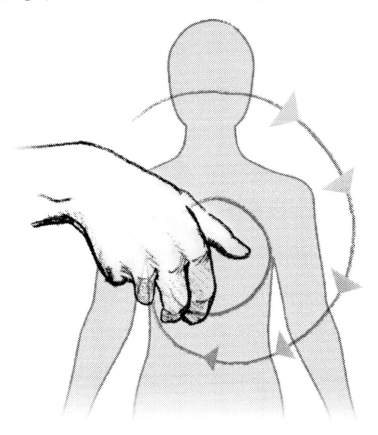

Clockwise Stirring.
The body is the face of the clock.

You may notice an area on one side or the other, on the top, or the bottom that is not as freely flowing. That is where you would want to focus extra attention.

A counter-clockwise motion can be used, but should be used cautiously. Many times counter-clockwise releases so much so quickly that the recipient feels unsettled or even nauseous. It is better to use counter-clockwise sparingly.

Exercise

Place your non-dominate hand over the first Chakra. With your dominate hand stir its energy in a <u>clockwise</u> direction for 8 to 10 revolutions while being aware of any imbalances (thickness, heaviness or slow moving). **Pause**. Now stir <u>counter-clockwise</u> 4 to 6 revolutions. **Pause**. Now stir again in a <u>clockwise</u> motion 8 to 10 revolutions.

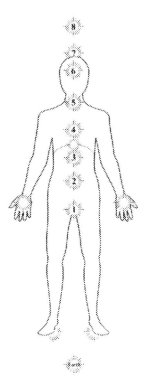

Remember this is not a race! Be gentle. Take the time you need to clear any stagnations.

What did you feel or sense? Does the energy feel clear and smooth, or does it need additional clearing?

If the energy needs additional clearing, repeat clockwise and the alternating counter-clockwise stirring until the energy feels smooth. Always end in a clockwise motion.

As you clear each chakra, **pause**. Gently move to the next chakra, connect and repeat the stirring technique. When you have completed stirring the chakras remember to gently disconnect.

Chapter Review

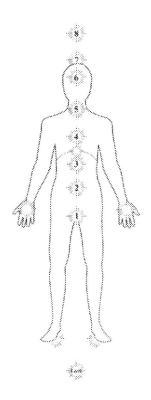

Chakras

The word Chakra is of Sanskrit origin (an ancient language of India) meaning vortex or spinning wheel.

These spinning energy centers are responsible for bringing in fresh energies for the body to use and removing stagnate, or used, energy from the body.

Each Chakra resonates at its own unique vibrational rate which is used to support the body systems it serves.

The core, or centers, of the major body Chakras are positioned along a column of energy that parallels the inside portion of the spine.

Chakras also imprint records of past traumatic events (physical, mental, emotional, and/or spiritual) in a person's life.

Stirring

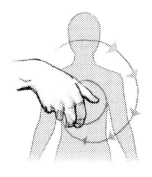

The stirring technique is a wonderful way to locate and clear stagnant energy within a sphere of energy.

When using the stirring technique visualize extending the energy from the ends of your fingers into a fishbowl. Use your energy fingers to gently stir the energy (within the bowl) in a clockwise motion.

While stirring focus your intention on any areas in the bowl of energy that may feel different from the rest. Continue to gently stir until all areas of the energy bowl feel clear and smooth.

Chapter 3

Energy Flow

"Your body is your subconscious mind,

and it controls your programs."

Unknown

<u>Energy is Movement</u>

Many techniques taught in various traditions of energy medicine teach you to hold one point with another until the points feel balanced.

What I want you to understand is that energy should be freely moving.

Helping energy to move freely in a fashion similar to the flow of a garden sprinkler or the dancing fountains at the Bellagio Hotel in Las Vegas is our first goal.

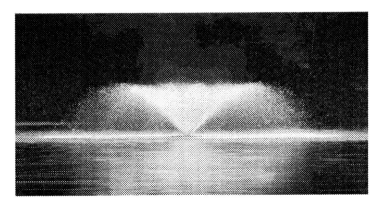

Move the energy upward, and then follow its return in the downward flow. With this movement, you connect with the inner and outer, the top and bottom, the front and the back, and the right and left of the energy.

The smooth flow of all portions of the energy is important for the health and well-being of each cell within our bodies. As we begin connecting and moving energy we want to keep this fact in the forefront of our awareness.

The Flow of Energy

Most of us have heard that there is a Yin and a Yang portion to energy.

The Yin and Yang of energy simply represent the natural dualities in our world. E.g. black and white, low and high, dark and light, male and female, hot and cold, left and right, <u>up and down</u>. The two cannot live without each other.

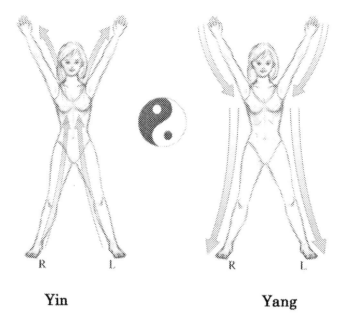

Yin

Yang

The Yin portion is the inner aspect and flows upward. It is associated with the left or feminine side of our body.

The Yang portion is the outer aspect and flows downward. It is associated with the right or masculine side of our body.

So the natural flow of energy is in a Yin (upward), and Yang (downward), motion - just like the flow of a fountain or garden sprinkler.

The drawing on the next page shows us how we can move energy in a fountain like movement by coming up in the core, opening up and then cascading back down to the base of the flow where it returns up again.

Our job is to pay attention to where this flow of energy is not freely moving. This can be a small portion on the upward flow or even a slice on the downward flow. For true harmony, we need all of the flow to be smooth.

Energy Flow Illustration

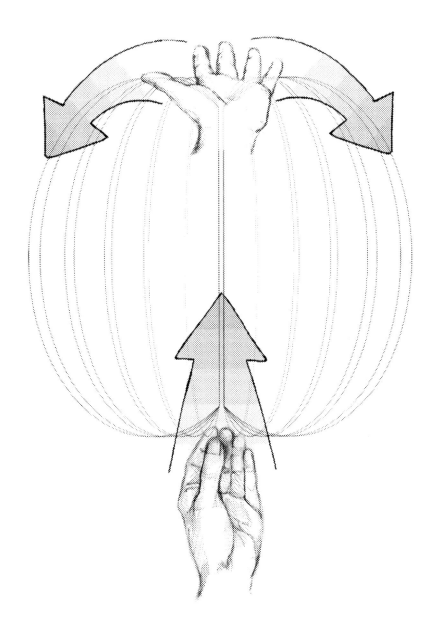

Energy flows upward through the center Yin flow and returns downward following the outside Yang flow. By repeating this Yin and Yang movement, we help restore balance throughout this energy fountain.

Grounding Points

Grounding points, also called the "Wellspring of Life Points", are the first point of the Kidney Meridian. It is said this meridian contains the life force of beginnings and renewal.

A person's grounding points are located on the bottom of the feet just below the ball of each foot. The grounding points may be located slightly differently on each foot and may also be located slightly differently on each client.

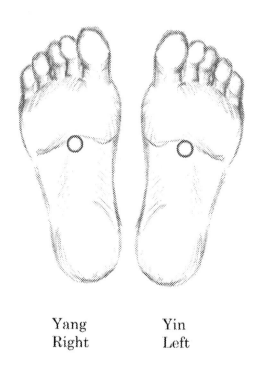

Yang   Yin
Right   Left

Why We Ground

Our physical body is sustained by the earth's energy. Our bones, muscles, connective tissue and organs throughout our entire body are supported by the earth's vibrational energy.

To keep our physical body functioning correctly, we need to keep it in harmony with the earth. We can do this for ourselves and others by connecting the grounding points with our earth chakra or the core of the earth.

Energy Flow

<u>Self-Grounding</u>

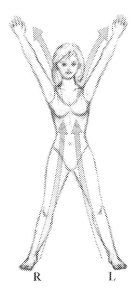

Here is a wonderful way to ground ourselves.

First energetically connect to your grounding points.

After you feel you have made a strong connection pull the energy up the inside of your legs.

Continue up the front of your body, and up inside your arms to the center of you palms.

Allow the energy to sit in your palms for a few moments.

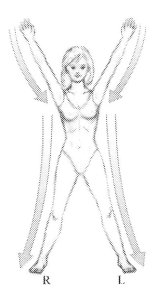

Now allow the energy to spill out the center of your palms.

Bring the energy down the outside of your arms and continuing down the sides of your body and legs to the bottom of your feet.

Feel the energy re-enter the bottoms of your feet.

Now repeat the upward and downward movements as above until all your energy feels smooth and grounded.

Grounding Exercises

Exercise - Energy Flow and the Grounding Points.

Remember, you are working in another person's energy. Always connect and disconnect to their energy gently!

Expand the flow

Center and focus yourself before you connect. Your focus at this time is to move the energy up thru the grounding point of the foot and back down the outside of the foot, and repeat.

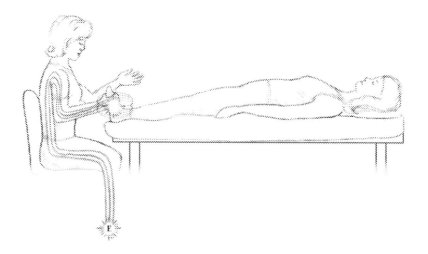

Connect your right hand to the grounding point of the left foot. Remember, the left side is the connection to the Yin or inner and upward flow of energy.

Now, with clarity of focus and intention, use your left hand to move the energy up thru the grounding point of the foot and back down the outside of the foot, and repeat.

Give yourself the opportunity to sense the energy. Is the energy running up and down? Are there any distortions? Be aware of the transitions up/down, down/up.

Now repeat the same technique with the client's right foot. When you have finished gently disconnect.

Energy Flow and Both Feet

Exercise - Energy flow and both grounding points.

Connect to the grounding points on both feet at the same time. With clarity of focus and intention, imagine having an extra set of hands and run the energy flow through the grounding points. Return it to the Earth and then back up to the grounding points.

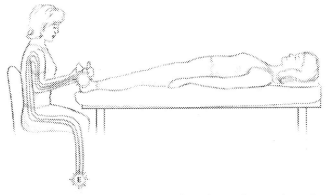

Practice until you are comfortable with the idea of running the energy flow without having to move the energy using your hands.
Gently disconnect.

Exercise - Energy flow, grounding points, Earth and the hips.

Connect to the grounding points on both feet at the same time. With clarity of focus and intention, bring energy flow up from the Earth, through the grounding points and up the inside of the legs to the hips. Return it down the outside of the legs, through the grounding points, to the Earth.

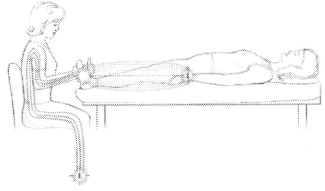

Repeat this process until the flow of energy feels balanced on both grounding points. Gently disconnect.

Full Body Energy Flow

The use of energy flow throughout the entire body is a very powerful way to clear disharmony when releasing congestion.

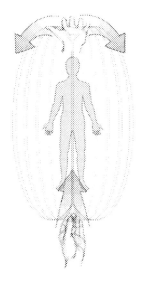

Exercise

While holding the grounding points, visualize energy flowing up through the core of the person, out of the top of their head, and outward to the edge of the body. Then return it downward to the Earth and back up to the grounding points.

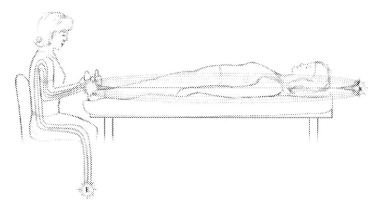

Repeat this Full Body Energy Flow until the upwards and downwards energy feels cleared. Gently disconnect.

Chapter Review

Energy Flow

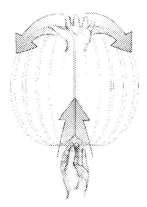

Remember that energy should be freely flowing, similar to the flow of a garden sprinkler or fountain. We want to move energy in a fountain like movement, coming up through the core. Then opening up and cascading back down to return to the base where the flow returns back up again.

Grounding Points

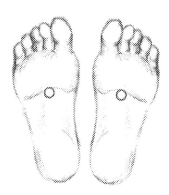

To keep our physical body functioning correctly we need to keep it in harmony with the earth. We can do this for ourselves and others by connecting the grounding points with the person's earth chakra or core of the earth.

Full Body Energy Flow

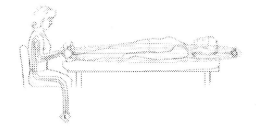

Visualize sending energy up through the core of the person and up through the top of their head. Then cascade back down and return to the person's earth chakra where the flow returns back up again.

45

Chapter 4

Energy Flow

and

Chakras

"The best way to find yourself,

is to lose yourself in

the service of others."

Mahatma Gandhi

Exercise

In this exercise we will be applying the Energy Flow technique to the Chakras. Using energy flow assists with an even bigger expansion of each chakra. This expansion allows a better flow of energy coming into the body and then releases more stagnate energy out of the body. With this better flow, the chakra can support more healing.

Gently place your non-dominate hand on the first Chakra. With your dominate hand use the energy flow technique to identify if the energy is stagnant, sluggish or out of balance. Continue to use energy flow until the Chakra feels smooth and balanced. Gently disconnect.

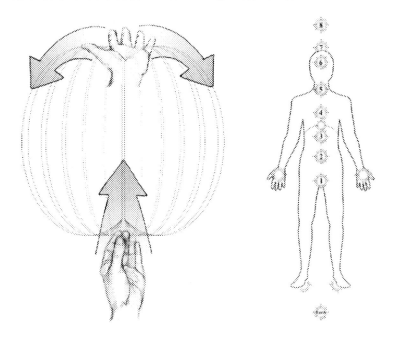

Gently place your non-dominate hand on the second Chakra and use energy flow. Does this Chakra feel smooth and balanced? Does the energy feel similar to the first Chakra? Use energy flow to clear any disharmony and restore balance. Gently disconnect.

Remember that each chakra has a unique vibration, so each chakra will most likely have a slightly different feel to it when in balance.

Repeat the same procedure with each of the other Chakras. Try to identify the difference in vibration for each Chakra, and remember to always <u>gently</u> connect and disconnect to each Chakra.

<u>Body Chakra Flow</u>

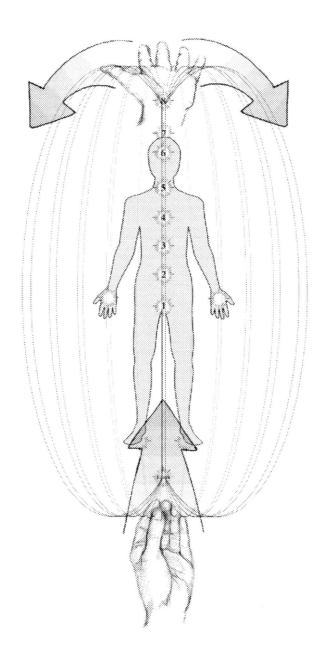

Using the Body Chakra Flow is a very powerful way to clear stagnations from the energy and balance the Chakras.

Body Chakra Flow

Exercise

During this Body Chakra Flow exercise we will send energy up to each of the individual chakras, expand it out, return it down to the Earth chakra and bring it back up to the grounding points.

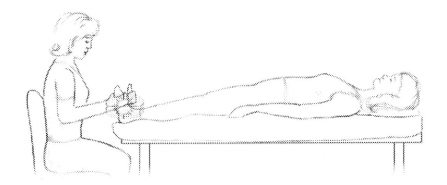

1 - Connect to the grounding points on both feet. With the clarity of focus and intention, balance both grounding points using energy flow.

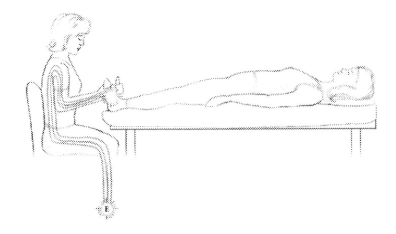

2 - While continuing to hold the grounding points, send the energy flow down to the Earth Chakra and connect. Return the energy up from the Earth Chakra to the grounding points. Notice any change in the flow. Repeat this procedure until the flow feels clear and balanced.

Body Chakra Flow (First & Second)

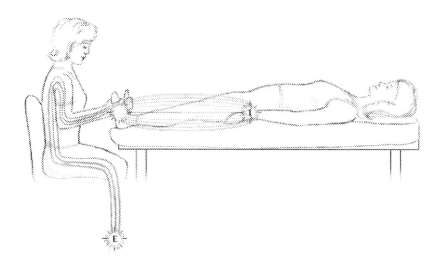

3 - Now bring the energy from the Earth Chakra up through the grounding points and legs to the First Chakra. Expand it outward and return it down on the outside of the legs, through the grounding points back down to the Earth Chakra. Repeat this procedure until the flow feels clear balanced.

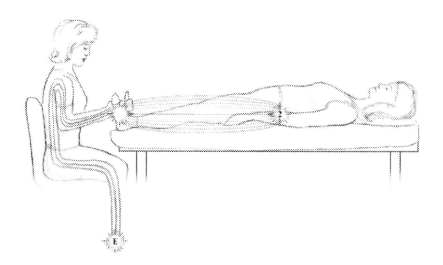

4 - Start the flow again at the Earth Chakra, moving it up through the grounding points, legs, First Chakra, and up to the Second Chakra. Expand the flow outward and return it down the outside of the legs, through the grounding points back to the Earth Chakra. Repeat this procedure until the flow feels clear and balanced.

Body Chakra Flow (Third & Forth)

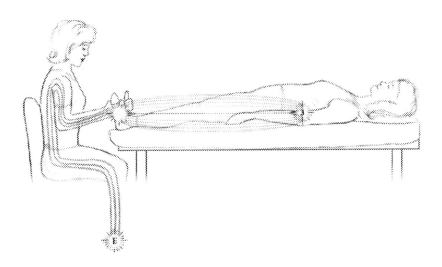

5 - Start the flow again at the Earth Chakra, moving it up through the grounding points, legs, First and Second Chakras to the Third Chakra. Expand the flow outward and return it back down outside the body, legs, through the grounding points down to the Earth Chakra. Repeat this procedure until the flow feels clear and balanced.

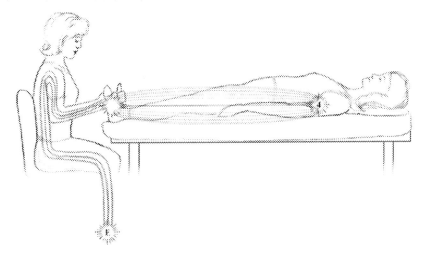

6 - Start the flow again at the Earth Chakra, move it up through the grounding points, legs, First, Second and Third Chakras to the Fourth Chakra. Expand the flow outward and return it back down outside the body, legs, through the grounding points down to the Earth Chakra. Repeat this procedure until the flow feels clear and balanced.

Body Chakra Flow (Fifth & Sixth)

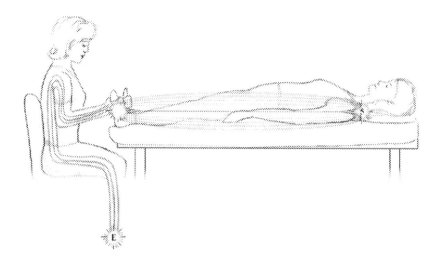

7 - Start the flow again at the Earth Chakra, move it up through the grounding points, legs, First, Second, Third and Forth Chakras to the Fifth Chakra. Expand the flow outward and return it back down outside the body, legs, through the grounding points down to the Earth Chakra. Repeat this procedure until the flow feels clear and balanced.

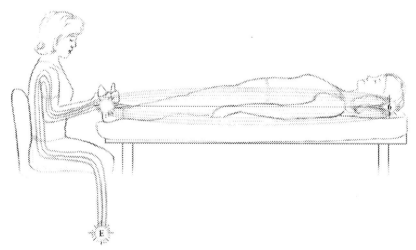

8 - Start the flow again at the Earth Chakra, move it up through the grounding points, legs, First, Second, Third, Forth and Fifth Chakras to the Sixth Chakra. Expand the flow outward and return it back down outside the body, legs, through the grounding points down to the Earth Chakra. Repeat this procedure until the flow feels clear and balanced.

Body Chakra Flow (Seventh & Eighth)

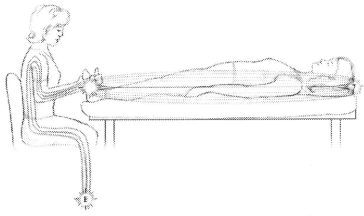

9 - Start the flow again at the Earth Chakra, move it up through the grounding points, legs and up the Chakras to the Seventh Chakra. Expand the flow outward and return it back down outside the body, legs, through the grounding points down to the Earth Chakra. Repeat this procedure until the flow feels clear and balanced.

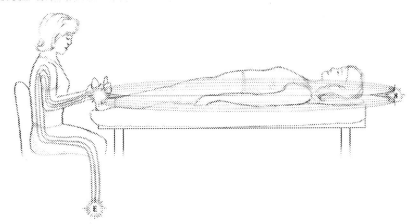

10 - Start the flow again at the Earth Chakra, move it up through the grounding points, legs and up the Chakras to the Eighth Chakra. Expand the flow outward and return it back down outside the body, legs, through the grounding points down to the Earth Chakra. Repeat this procedure until the flow feels clear and balanced.

You have now completed the Full Body Chakra Flow. This exercise can greatly open and balance the energy of the entire body. It is a wonderful technique to use on someone who does not have time for a full session. This technique can also give an assessment of where energy may not be moving well, and then you can address that specific area.

Chapter Review

Energy Flow with the Chakras

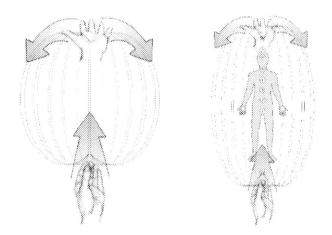

Applying the Energy Flow technique to the Chakras assists with a bigger expansion of each chakra. This expansion allows a better flow of energy coming into, and releases more stagnate energy out of, the body. With this better flow, each chakra can support more healing.

Full Body Chakra Flow

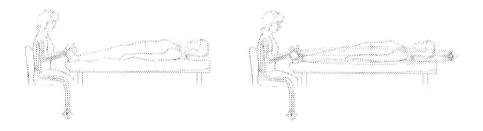

Connect to the grounding points. Send the energy up to each individual chakra, expand it out and return it down to the earth chakra. Repeat this process for each chakra until you have cleared all eight chakras.

Chapter 5

Expanding

Energy Flow

"Sometimes your joy is the source of your smile,

but sometimes

your smile can be the source of your joy."

Thich Nhat Hanh

Energy Aspects

As we continue the journey into this wonderful world of energy healing, we will expand your knowledge on ways to connect, clear and balance energy systems.

Let's begin with a brief look at the unique **aspects** of energy.

The definition of <u>aspect</u>: the appearance of something from a specific viewpoint or perspective.

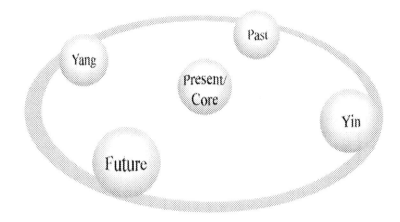

The Five Aspects of Energy Represent

- **Present/Core**   central portion
- **Yin**   feminine or inner portion
- **Yang**   masculine or outer portion
- **Future**   restrictions projected into your future
- **Past**   energies still held in past events

Remembering that all energies have these aspects can help you clarify your focus and intention when clearing stagnation. This clarified focus can facilitate clearing deeper levels of held disharmonies.

By releasing these deeper levels, you will greatly assist your clients in achieving greater improvements in their daily lives.

<u>Energy Perspectives</u>

Perspective – a specific point of view in understanding events.

The perspective changes depending on your point of view.

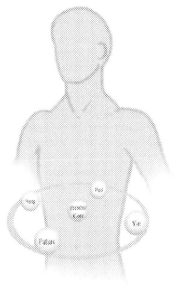

Your aspects as you would view them:

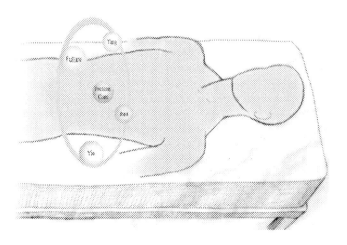

A client's aspects as viewed by you:

As you begin a session, remember to focus your intention on the correct perspective of the person's energy you are working on.

Introduction to the Wheel of Energy

As we see below, one of the better known wheels of energy is the Native American Medicine Wheel. This wheel has a core, or center, and four primary directions, or aspects. This wheel is used to assist people in strengthening their connection to the many aspects of Mother Nature and to create a stronger connection to their own strengths.

THE MEDICINE WHEEL

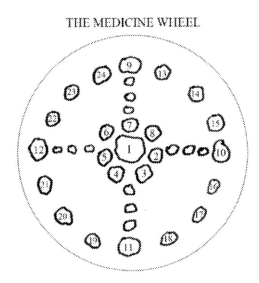

The major points of the Medicine Wheel radiate out from the center to the four primary directions – North, East, South and West. Each of the four directions are connected to two of the other directions as well as the center of the wheel.

Each of the directions is associated with specific nature elements, power animals and personal strengths. Each nature element may also vary depending upon the specific tribe.

The Four Directions

North	**East**	**South**	**West**
Elders	Children	Youth	Parents
Bear	Eagle	Wolf	Buffalo
Cedar	Tobacco	Sweetgrass	Sage
Winter	Spring	Summer	Fall
Wind	Fire	Earth	Water

The Energy Wheel

We will be using the Energy Wheel, as seen below, to help us connect to various aspects of specific energy.

When you sense or feel that a specific energy does not feel balanced (see page 21), check each of the aspects to see if they are out of balance.
By restoring balance to each aspect, you restore harmony to the specific energy.

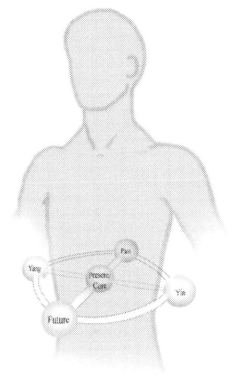

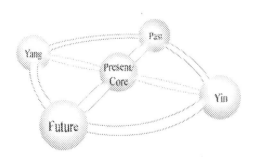

The Energy Wheel helps us locate where a specific energy's imbalance is being held so we can focus the clearing to that area.

Exercise - The Energy Wheel at the Chakras

Start by placing the Energy Wheel on the Earth Chakra. Use Energy Flow on each aspect (The Core, Yin, Yang, Future and Past) and clear its energy. Focus your awareness to sense how the aspects compare. **Pause.**

Now use the Stirring technique on each of the aspects (The Core, Yin, Yang, Future and Past) and clear its energy. Again focus your awareness to sense how each aspect compares. **Pause.**

Continue repeating this same process to as many of the chakras as time allows. Once finished, ask your practice partner if they noticed any difference in the work at the beginning (Energy Flow) compared to the ending (Stirring) of each chakra.

Flowing 8

The Flowing 8 is also known as the infinity sign which has neither a beginning nor ending. The Flowing 8 is also seen in the Caduceus, the intertwined serpents found on the staff that is the symbol of the medical profession.

Since the body's energies spin, spiral, curve, crisscross and vibrate at different frequencies, we need a way to weave our energy fields and energetic structures together in various directions.

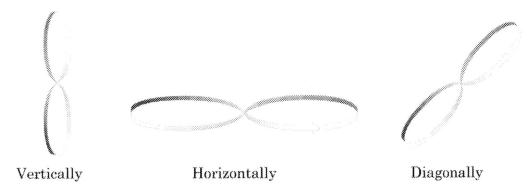

Vertically   Horizontally   Diagonally

The Flowing 8 can lace through your energy systems and help create a resonance among them. When we have resonance between our energy systems, information can easily travel wherever it needs to go enabling all our energy systems to work in harmony.

Exercise - Flowing 8 on Wheel at the Chakras

Using the Flowing 8, connect and balance the energy between the Present/Core, of a selected Chakra and each of that Chakra's other aspects (Future, Yang, Past and Yin).

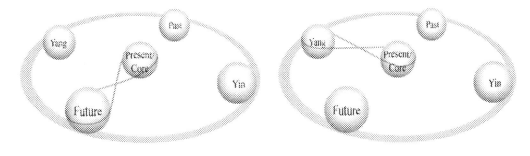

Present/Core + Future   Present/Core + Yang

Be sure each aspect feels clear and balanced before moving to the next aspect.

63

Flowing 8 with Wheel

Exercises

Continue to balance the Present/Core <u>individually</u> with the other two outer aspects.

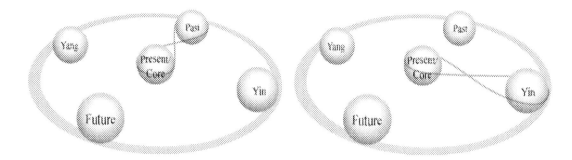

Present/Core + Past   Present/Core + Yin

Once you have completed balancing the Present/Core with each of the outer aspects shift your intention to balance the outer aspects with each other.

Place the center of the Flowing 8 in the Present/Core and flow outward to the Yin aspect back through the Core outward to the Yang aspect and back to the Core.

Continue this movement until the energy feels clear and balanced. Then use the same technique to clear and balance the Future and Past aspects.

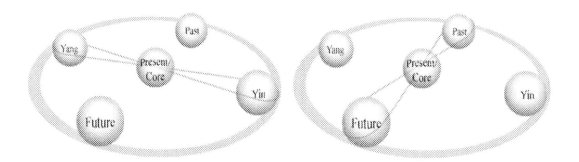

Yin & Yang <u>thru</u> the Present/Core.   Future & Past <u>thru</u> the Present/Core.

The Flowing 8 can also be used to balance the energy between each of the outer aspects (Yin with Future, Yin with Past, Yang with Future, Yang with Past, etc.).

Expanded Energy Wheel

As we continue to expand ways to clear and balance disharmonies within energy systems, let us look at how to expand the information supplied by the Energy Wheel.

We know Energy Wheels exist within other vibrations. There are frequencies that are higher in vibration (which does not mean better) and frequencies that are lower in vibration (which does not mean less important).

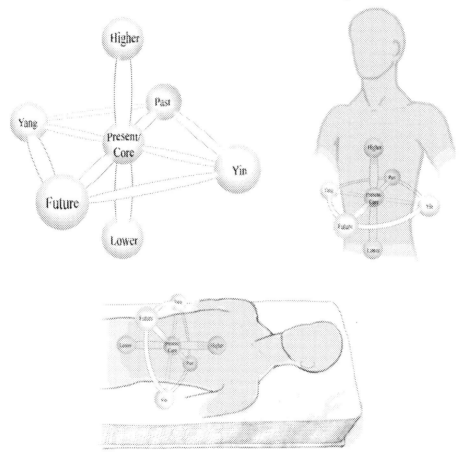

So we can bring more harmony to the system or area we are working on, let's expand the Energy Wheel to connect with these higher and lower vibrations.

From the core of the wheel, extend upward to the next closest vibration and then downward to the next closest vibration.

You now have the expanded Energy Wheel.

The Pyramid

The Pyramid is the fully expanded version of the Energy Wheel.

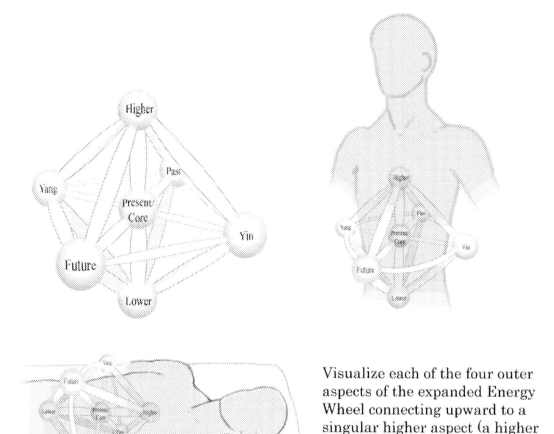

Visualize each of the four outer aspects of the expanded Energy Wheel connecting upward to a singular higher aspect (a higher vibration).

Next visualize each of the four outer aspects also connecting downward to a singular lower aspect (a lower vibration).

When using the Pyramid, envision the flow coming up through the lower aspect, through the Present/Core, to the higher aspect. The energy then cascades down through the outer aspects of the wheel returning to the lower aspect of the Pyramid.

Remember - Energy Flow!

Expanding Energy Flow

The Pyramid Exercise

The Pyramid may be used to clear and or connect energies of chakras, organs, joints or various areas of the body.

In this exercise, we will be using the Pyramid to clear and balance energies within the chakras.

Exercise

Connect to the First Chakra.

Place the Pyramid Core on the Chakra's Core, and the Pyramid's *Above* aspect connecting to the Core of the Second Chakra and the Pyramid's *Below* aspect connecting to the Core of the Earth Chakra.

Using the Flowing 8, balance the energy between the Pyramid's Core and each of it's other aspects - Future, Yin, Past, Yang, Higher (Core of the higher chakra) and Lower (Core of the lower chakra).

Be sure each aspect feels clear and balanced before moving to the next aspect. Once you have completed balancing the Pyramids Core with each of its outer aspects, shift your intention to balance the Pyramids outer aspects with each other.

Start the Flowing 8 in the center of the Core and flow to the Yin, then back through the Core to the Yang and return to the Core. Continue this movement until the energy feels clear and balanced.

Using the same technique, clear and balance the Future and Past aspects.

Continuing this same technique, clear and balance the Higher and Lower aspects until the energy of the Pyramid is in harmony.

Move the Pyramid to the Second Chakra with the *Above* aspect connecting to the Core of the Third Chakra and the *Below* aspect connecting to the Core of the First Chakra. Using the same technique, clear and balance all aspects of this new Chakra Pyrimid.

Repeat the process until you have harmonized as many Chakras as time allows.

The Paddle

When working with various energies, there are times when a larger mass of energy may be very stagnate, thick or sluggish. When this type of energy is found, the "Paddle" is a very useful tool to break up the stagnate area.

Envision a paddle, like a broad mixing spatula on a shaft which is rotated in three different directions to help break up heavy stagnation.

The three directions of the Paddle's movement are illustrated below.

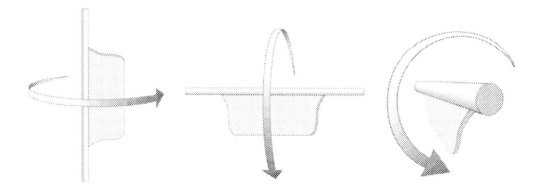

Shaft is vertical.   Shaft is left to right.   Shaft is front to back.

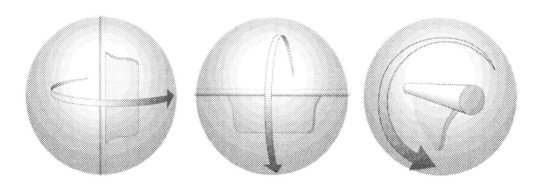

The Paddle shown in a sphere of stagnate energy.

The Paddle Continued

The difference between Stirring and The Paddle:

Stirring
        Used in clockwise or counter clockwise directions.
        Used more for releasing emotional stagnations.
        Areas that are <u>not</u> in a physically heavy stagnation.

Paddle:
        Used in left to right side rotation
        Used in a downward and upward rotation
        <u>Only</u> used in a counter clockwise direction
        For areas that are physically heavily stagnated

Exercise

Connect to a stagnate area with your non-dominant hand. Envision the paddle with its shaft in a vertical position centered within the stagnant area. You may also use your hand to represent the paddle movement.

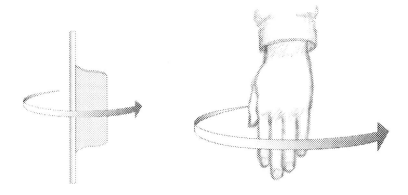

With your thoughts or dominant hand move the leading edge of the paddle in a counter clockwise movement. Starting at the left side, around the front to the right side, and return on the back portion to the left side. Repeat this rotation for four to six rotations. **Pause**.

Does the energy feel better or does it need additional rotations? Repeat the procedure until the energy moves freely.

Paddle Exercise Continued

Pivot the paddle so the shaft is positioned from left to right within the stagnant area.

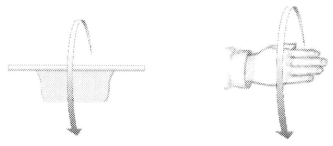

With your thoughts or dominant hand, rotate the paddle from the back over the top, down the front, under the bottom and back up the back. Repeat this rotation for four to six rotations.　**Pause**.

Does the energy feel better or does it need additional rotations? Repeat the procedure until the energy moves freely.

Now pivot the paddle so the shaft is positioned from front to back within the stagnant area.

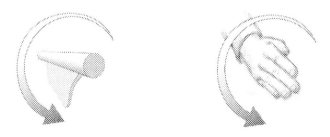

With your thoughts or dominant hand, rotate the paddle from the top, down the left side, under the bottom and up the right side to the top. Repeat this rotation for four to six rotations.　**Pause**.

Does the energy feel better or does it need additional rotations? Repeat the procedure until the energy moves freely.

If the energy was very thick or sluggish, repeat all three rotation positions until the entire area is flowing easily.

Chapter Review

Aspects

The appearance of something from a specific viewpoint of perspective.

Energy Aspects

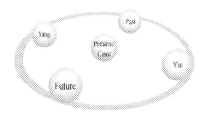

Present/Core — central portion

Yin – feminine or inner portion
    (left side of the energy)

Yang – masculine or outer portion
    (right side of the energy)

Future – restrictions projected into your future
    (front side of the energy)

Past – energies still held in past events
    (back side of the energy)

Energy Wheel

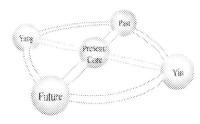

The Energy Wheel helps us connect to five aspects of the specific energy we are working with. Each of the Wheel's aspects connect to the center and to each other.

Remember that all energies have the above aspects, and the Wheel can help you clarify your focus and intention when clearing stagnation to bring balance and harmony.

Flowing 8

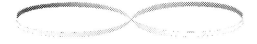

The Flowing 8 is also known as the infinity sign which has neither a beginning nor ending. Since the body's energies spin, spiral, curve, crisscross and vibrate at different frequencies we use the Flowing 8 to weave our energy fields and energetic structures together.

Chapter Review Continued

Pyramid

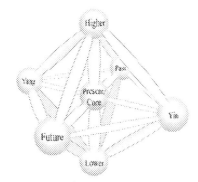

The pyramid is an expanded version of the Energy Wheel. The pyramid adds a higher and lower aspect which allows you to expand the energies you're working with. For example, you can connect the core of one Chakra and connect it to the core of a higher vibrational Chakra and to the core of the lower vibrational Chakra.

Paddle

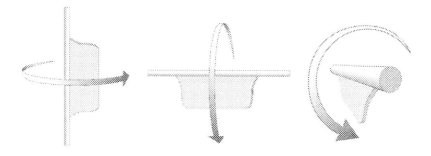

The paddle is a tool that is like a broad mixing spatula, on a shaft, which is rotated in three different directions. The paddle can be used to break up heavy, stagnate, thick or sluggish energy anywhere in the body.

Chapter 6

Gateways

to

Emotions

"Each organ and gland

has its own unique energy vibration.

Our goal is to get them

to play together in harmony."

Bruce Winkle

Introduction

The word emotion comes from a Latin verb which literally means "energy in motion." What we think of as emotion is the experience of energy moving through our body.

Emotional energy is neutral, but it is the feeling sensations and our physiological reactions that give the energy meaning. Emotions serve as a carrier for our entire spectrum of feelings.

Our emotions are a natural part of our existence that allows us to experience life. While the power of positive emotions can enrich our lives, the power of negative emotions can just as easily destroy us.

Examples of positive emotions include- joy, happiness, love and inner peace.

Examples of negative emotions include – anger, fear, hate and unresolved grief.

Our emotions play a vital role in creating the internal energy in our organs, muscles, chakras, tissue and meridians that lead to both health and disease.

Gateways

Gateways are the access points to held emotional traumas.

We use the word Gateways because we are using organ connection points as a means to access the emotions that are held throughout the body.

Though each organ is associated with a selection of emotions, these emotions are not just located in the organ, they are held within cells throughout the body.

By connecting to these points, we have a greater ability to release the specifically trapped emotions held within all cells.

So let us begin our exploration into these wonderful Gateways with a brief review of the organs and their locations.

The emotions interconnected with each of the organs are listed on page 78.

Front View of Organs

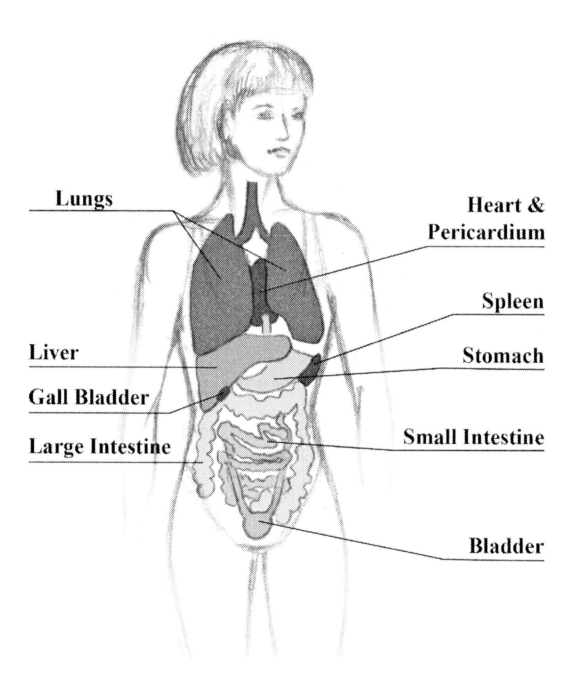

Lungs

Heart &
Pericardium

Spleen

Liver

Stomach

Gall Bladder

Large Intestine

Small Intestine

Bladder

The organs as viewed from the front.

Back View of Organs

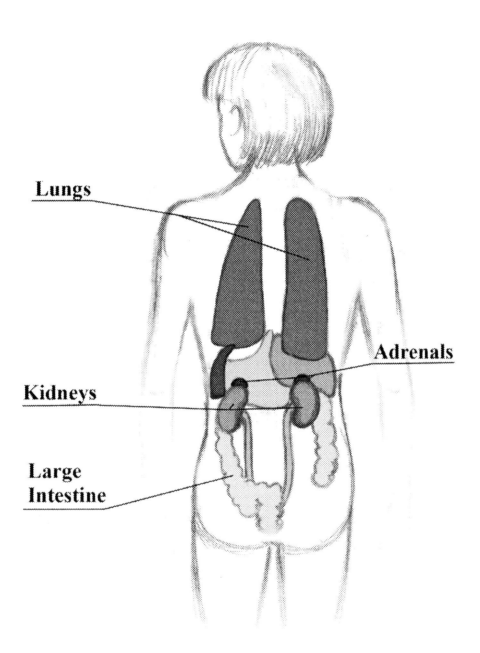

Lungs

Adrenals

Kidneys

Large Intestine

The organs as viewed from the back.

Emotions of the Organs

Organs are either known as Yin energy (inner and upward flowing) or Yang energy (outer and downward flowing). A deeper understanding of the Yin and Yang energies will be explored in the Pathways of Emotion course.

Kidneys (Yin)
> Fear, Shame, Guilt, Broken Will

Pericardium (Yin)
> Guarded, Inhibition, Greed, Tightness in the Chest

Adrenals (Yang)
> On Edge

Gallbladder (Yang)
> Resentment, Frustration, Cannot take Action

Liver (Yin)
> Anger, Blaming, Manipulation

Lungs (Yin)
> Grief, Chronic Sadness, Overcritical

Large Intestine (Yang)
> Unable to let Go, Feeling Trapped, Dogmatic, Compulsive

Stomach (Yang)
> Anxiety, Self-Punishment, Broken Power

Spleen (Yin)
> Low Self-Worth, Obsession

Heart (Yin)
> Lack of Joy, Loneliness, Acute Grief, Humiliation

Small Intestine (Yang)
> Insecure, Unworthy, Unlovable, Trapped

Bladder (Yang)
> Timidity, Shyness, Helplessness, Deep Exhaustion

Energetic Levels of Emotions

Lowest Levels of emotional energy are shame, guilt, apathy, and grief.

When energy is operating at these levels, there are usually multiple issues and problems causing the energetic imbalance throughout the body.

At this emotional level, it will take time and multiple treatments to clear and rebalance the person's system.

Middle Levels of emotional energy are fear, desire, anger, and pride.

At this middle level of emotional energy, it is possible for people to have a healthier life than at the lower level of energy.

However, this level has its own particular concerns. Many imbalances can be held in the body creating multiple health concerns as we travel on our journey.

Higher Levels include courage, neutrality, willingness, and acceptance.

This level is the beginning of a crossover point, where self power – rather than force – is used to make decisions and create change in your life.

At this level, there is a realization that our own empowerment and the empowerment of others are the true keys to success.

Exercise

Locate the twelve major organs and identify the related emotions.

When you are able, work with a partner on this exercise. One person will say the organ and the emotion that is held by that organ. The other person should locate the organ on their own body. Once finished, switch roles and repeat the same exercise with your partner.

The goal here is to become familiar with the location of the major organs and which emotion is associated with that organ.

The Gateways

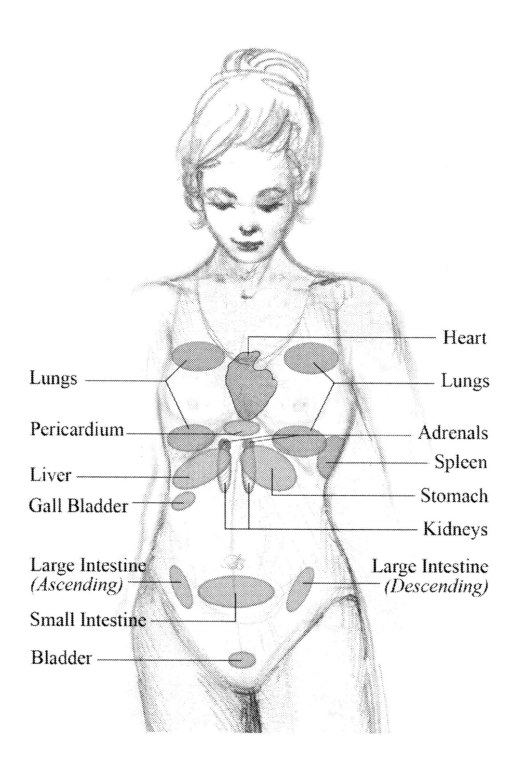

Heart

Lungs

Lungs

Pericardium

Adrenals

Spleen

Liver

Stomach

Gall Bladder

Kidneys

Large Intestine
(Ascending)

Large Intestine
(Descending)

Small Intestine

Bladder

Locations

Kidneys

 Accessed on either side of the spine at the bottom of the ribs.

Pericardium

 Approximately one inch below the bottom of the sternum.

Adrenals

 Accessed on top of the kidneys.

Gallbladder

 Accessed on the right side of the body approximately three inches below the end of the 11th rib (also known as floating rib).

Liver

 Accessed on the front of the body just below the right rib cage.

Lungs

 On the right side of the body, the lungs have three lobes. The upper lobe can be accessed just above the breasts; the middle lobe can be located on the side of the ribs; and the third lobe is just below the breast.
 The left side of the body only has two lobes. The upper lobe can be accessed above the breast, and the lower lobe is below the breast.

Large Intestines

 The start of the large intestines is the ascending portion which is accessed on the right side of the body just inside the pelvic girdle. The descending portion is accessed on the left side of the body just inside the pelvic girdle.

Stomach

 Accessed on the front of the body just below the left rib cage.

Spleen

 Accessed on the left side of the body at the lowest portion of the rib cage.

Heart

 May be accessed by laying your hand directly over the sternum. If this connection is uncomfortable for you or your client, you may access the Heart points on either side of the sternum in the space between the fourth and fifth ribs.

Small Intestines

 Accessed about two inches below the navel.

Bladder

 Accessed on the center line of the body just above the pubic bone.

Exercises

Exercise - Connecting to the Gateways

Start by placing a hand on the first Gateway and use Energy Flow to assess the energy within that Gateway. Proceed to connect with each of the twelve Gateways using Energy Flow to assess the energy of each one. Remember to connect to each Gateway when they are in pairs (example – Kidneys).
You may use your free hand to help you with Energy Flow or you may do it intuitively.

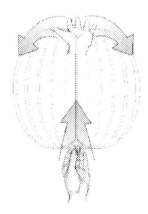

Exercise - Clearing the Gateways with Stirring and the Energy Wheel

Start by placing your non-dominant hand on the first Gateway and use Stirring to get a better sense of its energy. If you find stagnate energy within the Gateway, use the Energy Wheel to find the aspect of the Gateway that is holding the stagnation. Now use Stirring on that aspect to clear the stagnation.
Proceed through as many Gateways as possible in the time allowed.

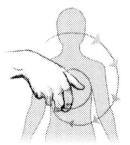
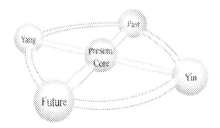

Exercises

Exercise - Connecting the Gateways with Flowing 8

Start by connecting to the Kidney Gateway and get a sense of its energy. Using your other hand, connect to the Pericardium Gateway. Now with focus and intention, use the Flowing 8 to balance the energy between the Kidney and the Pericardium Gateways.

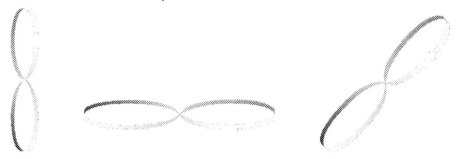

When the energy feels balanced between them, shift your attention from the Kidney to the Adrenal. With focus and intention use the Flowing 8 to balance the energy between the Pericardium and Adrenal Gateways.

When the energy feels balanced between them, move your hand from the Pericardium to the Gall Bladder. With focus and intention use the Flowing 8 to balance the energy between the Adrenal and Gall Bladder Gateways.

Continue to connect to each of the Gateways, in the following order, until you have finished balancing the energy between all twelve.

1-Kidney + Pericardium	2-Pericardium + Adrenal
3-Adrenal + Gall Bladder	4-Gall Bladder + Liver
5-Liver + Lungs	6-Lungs + Large Intestine
7-Large Intestine + Stomach	8-Stomach + Spleen
9-Spleen + Heart	10-Heart + Small Intestine
11-Small Intestine + Bladder	12-Bladder + Kidney

Remember to do <u>both</u> organs when organs are located on both sides of the body. (Kidneys, Adrenals, Lungs, Large Intestine)

The Gateways

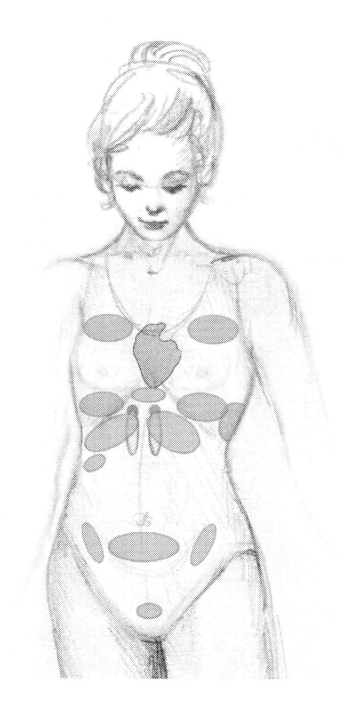

Use this illustration of the Gateways to practice identifying each one.

Chapter Review

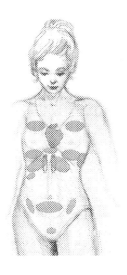

Organs

We learned the emotions associated with the 12 major organs. This knowledge helps us know which Gateway to work with when helping our clients release emotional traumas.

The 12 Gateways

Kidney, Pericardium, Adrenals, Gall Bladder.

Liver, Lungs, Large Intestines, Stomach.

Spleen, Heart, Small Intestines, Bladder.

The Energetic Levels of Emotions

Lowest Levels

Shame, guilt, apathy, and deep grief.

Middle Levels

Fear, desire, anger, and pride.

Higher Levels

Courage, neutrality, willingness, and acceptance.

Practice

Locating and connecting to each of the Gateways.

Chapter 7

Energies

of the

Heart

"When you place your awareness

in your heart,

you will naturally dwell in the

synchronicities of now."

Peggy Black

Our Heart

*"To heal the Heart is to become a balancing point
between Heaven and Earth".*

Most people are aware that their heart is the center of their circulatory system, carrying blood to over 75 trillion cells throughout their body. But our hearts play a much more powerful role in our bodies and lives.

Our heart is one of the body's major endocrine glands, producing at least five major hormones which impact the functions of the brain and body.

Our heart starts beating even before our brain has been formed. Within 20 days after conception our heart starts to function. The base of the brain does not function until around <u>90</u> days.

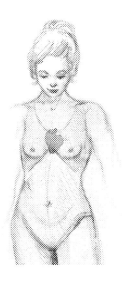

Our heart can act independently of the cranial brain and has extensive sensory capacities. In fact, between 60 and 65 percent of the heart cells are neural, identical to those present in the brain.

These heart cells are tightly organized, thus generating an extremely strong, intense and shared signal which is stronger than any other signal produced by any other part of the body. Thus the heart can dynamically move into the lead position in the body, its rhythms able to modulate or direct those of the other organs.

Information carried within energy waves flows constantly between the heart and the brain, assisting with our emotional processing, sensory experiences, our memory, and the meaning we derive from events. The heart sends more information to the brain than the brain sends to the heart.

<u>Our Heart</u>

*"The Heart governs the blood and pulse
as well as the mind and spirit".*

Our Heart is also the electromagnetic center of the body. The heart's electromagnetic field (EMF) is five thousand times stronger than that of the brain. Its electrical field is sixty times greater than that of the brain.

What about the heart's relationship with the external world?

We are constantly receiving information – sometimes called "background noise" – from outside of our inner selves. Most people believe that the brain initiates the first response to incoming events and then orders our reactions. Analysis reveals, however, that incoming information first impacts the heart, then travels through the heart, the brain and then rest of the body.

Not only can the heart override the incoming flow of communiqués, but it can also sort and filter information from the world outside of the body – even intuitive information.

Heart disease is the leading cause of death of American women, killing more than a third of them. Five times as many women die from heart attacks each year than from breast cancer. More women than men die of heart disease each year.

Heart disease is also the leading cause of death of American men, causing one in every four deaths. Between 70% and 89% of sudden cardiac events occur in men. Half of the men who die suddenly of coronary heart disease have no previous symptoms.

The National Coalition for Women with Heart Disease estimates 42 million American women live with cardiovascular disease, but too many are unaware of the threat they face.

Seeing how important the heart is to our entire life let's take a look at how we can help unlock our heart's healing power.

<u>The Heart</u>

Our Heart is the center of our body, as well as the home of our soul.

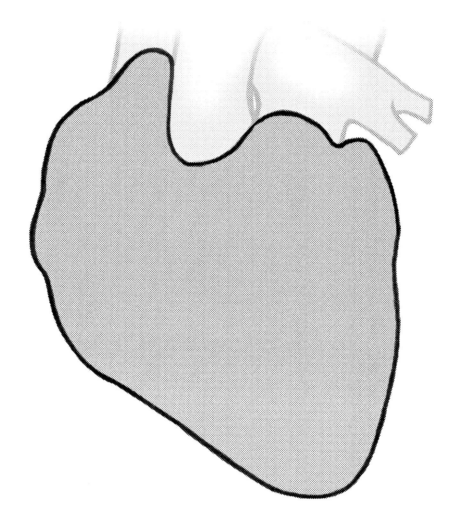

When a person consciously "centers" in their heart, the heart begins to direct the brain. Management of the body through the heart rather than brain leads us to higher levels of mental and emotional states, as well as healthier bodies.

<u>Fields of the Heart</u>

"Wherever your heart is, that is where you'll find your treasure."

Paulo Coelho

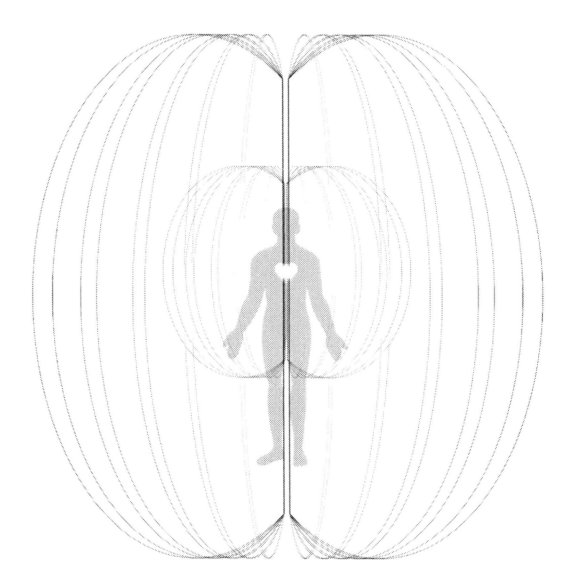

The electromagnetic and electrical fields change
according to the emotions we are holding in our hearts.

Fields of the Heart II

The heart produces larger electromagnetic and electrical fields than produced by the brain. With these larger fields, the heart can override, sort and filter the information we receive from the world including intuitive messages.

If positivity resides in our heart, it will attune to positivity. If fear, greed or anger resides within our heart, it will attune to negativity.

We can choose what our Hearts attune to!

Exercise

Visualize the Fields of the Heart as 12 layers.

Imagine each layer to be approximately 12"thick (in reality the thickness of each layer will vary depending upon its current condition). As a layer becomes clearer, it will expand. Each layer is unique unto its self.

You may connect coming up the sternum from the body or slide over the shoulder. If you come over the shoulder, be sure to **touch the shoulder first** before connecting to the heart to let the person know where you are.

Begin each session with connecting and grounding your client.

Gently place your hand on the body and then move gently to the Heart and connect. Take a few moments to just be with its energy before you begin any work. Since this is very deep work, it is a nice to place your other hand on the persons arm to add additional support to the clearing.

Start with the 12th layer, and clear each layer working inward toward the Heart.

Clear each layer using the Paddle. Use the Paddle in all three directions and repeat until the layer feels clear and expanded.

When you feel the layer is clear and vibrant, move inward to the next layer and repeat the procedure.

Clear as many layers as time will allow.

Layers of the Heart

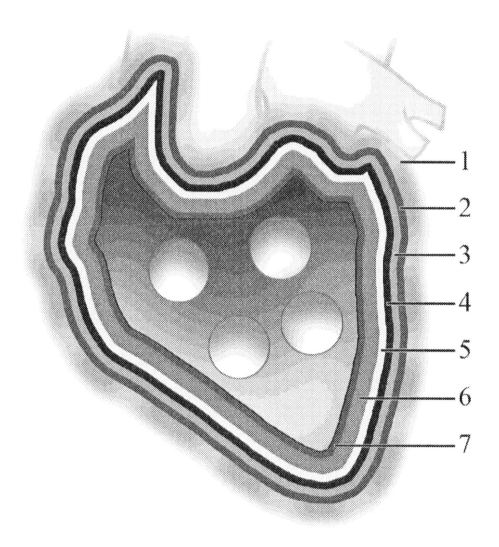

Most of us think of the heart as a layer of muscle with four chambers, miscellaneous valves, some arteries and veins, all surrounded by a sack called the pericardium.

But the structure of the heart is more involved, and we will now learn why and how it can become cut off from the rest of the body.

As we continue our study of the Heart, we will look at the layers that surround it and the make-up of its physical structure.

<u>Heart Layer Descriptions</u>

1 – Inner aspect of the electromagnetic field.
    This inner layer of the electromagnetic field communicates directly with the pericardium supplying a continual flow of information from the external world to the heart, and from the heart back to the world.

2 - Fibrous Pericardium -
    This outer most layer of the pericardium is made up of dense and loose connective tissue which anchor and protect the heart.

3 - Parietal Pericardium -
    The outer layer of the double wall sac containing the pericardial fluid.

4 - Pericardial Cavity -
    This is space between the parietal and the epicardium which contains the supply of the pericardial fluid.

5 – Epicardium – Also known as the Visceral Layer.
    The outer layer of the heart tissue and also the inner layer of the pericardium. It produces the pericardium fluid which lubricates motion between the inner and outer layers of the pericardium.

6 – Myocardium –
    The thick cardiac muscle of the heart which forms the foundation of the working heart.

7 – Endocardium –
    The innermost layer of tissue that lines the chambers of the heart which provides protection to the valves and chambers.

Note: When working on the layers, begin at the <u>outer</u> layer, #1 (which is the inner layer of the field) and work inward to layer #7.

Stirring the Heart

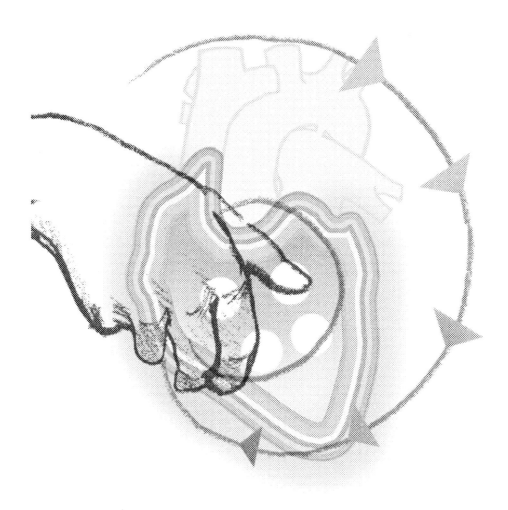

Stir each layer of the heart in a <u>clockwise</u> movement, as shown above, for four to six revolutions. Remember, **do not** stir in a counter clockwise motion! The counter clockwise movement could bring up many issues at a single time and probably over whelm the person and possibly yourself.

The heart is the face of the clock with;
12 o'clock at the top,
3 o'clock on the Yin side,
6 o'clock at the bottom and,
9 o'clock on the Yang side.

Stirring the Heart II

Note about the layers.

As you may have noticed, the first five layers of the heart have to do with protection. The longer a heart has been locked in protection or survival **mode**, the thicker and more resistant a layer will be to fully relax and release its held traumas.

By repeating the exercise below on a regular basis (on yourself and your clients), the more open and stronger the heart will become.

Exercise

Connect gently with the Heart.

Do not rush into the exercise, but allow a quiet moment of connection between your hearts.

Now visualize and connect to the 1st or outer layer of the client's Heart.

Gently begin stirring this layer, <u>clockwise</u>, for 10 to 12 revolutions. Pay close attention to each portion of the revolution. If a specific revolution is stagnant or begins to release lots of stored issues, stir that revolution until it clears before continuing with the remaining revolutions.

If you encountered stagnations and/or wonderful releases in a specific layer repeat stirring that layer with 10 to 12 more revolutions to be sure the layer is truly clear.

If a specific layer contains intense releasing, **<u>Pause</u>** for a few moments and then gently begin on that layer again. If it is still intensely releasing, **<u>Pause,</u>** and then move back 1 or more layers and begin again.

When you feel you have cleared a specific layer, move inward to the next layer and repeat this procedure.

When you have completed clearing the seven layers as much as possible for this session, remain connected to the Heart for a few minutes to support any ongoing clearing. Then <u>gently</u> disconnect from the Heart.

Chambers of the Heart

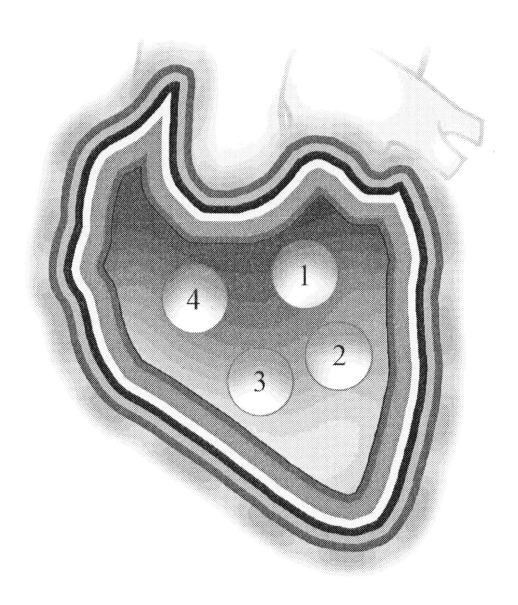

1 · Physical –   Relates to the nature and all matter

2 · Mental –   Relates to the mind or intellect

3 · Emotional – Relates to a strong feeling

4 · Energetic – Relates to the basis of all life

Chambers of the Heart Exercise

As the Heart vibrates so does the blood that flows through it.

The chambers lay within the seven layers of the Heart. They are the portals through which the blood is moved from the body to the lungs, and from the lungs back into the rest of the body.

Exercise

The Chambers relate to many aspects of our being, so we will use the Pyramid to clear each one.

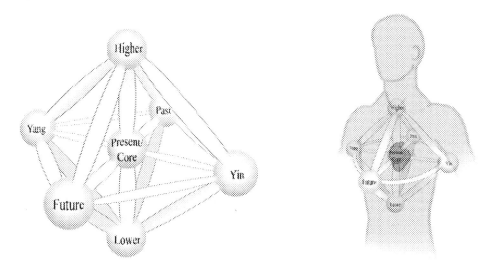

Begin by connecting to the first Chamber, the upper Yin side, of the Heart.

Place a Pyramid over the chamber and begin clearing each aspect using Energy Flow and/or Stirring. After clearing each of the aspects connect all the aspects using the Flowing 8 until the Pyramid feels vibrant over this Chamber

Now shift your awareness and connection to the second Chamber, the lower Yin side, of the Heart. Repeat clearing this chamber using the Pyramid as above.

Using the Pyramid, clear the third Chamber, the lower Yang side and then the fourth Chamber, the upper Yang side, to complete the session.

Connecting Heart Layers and Chakras

Since the Heart is connected with the events in our journeys, it is a wonderful clearing to connect each of the heart's layers with each of the seven primary chakras.

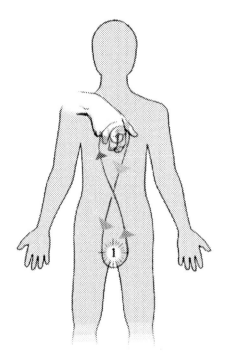

Exercise

In this exercise, we will be connecting and clearing <u>each</u> layer of the heart with each Chakra.

Begin by gently connecting to heart with one hand and the 1st Chakra with your other hand. Stir the first layer three to five times. Then using the Flowing 8, (vertically) connect the heart with the Chakra. Flow with this connection four to six (or more) times until the connection feels clear and vibrant. **Pause.**

Repeat this procedure with each heart layer. Be sure to notice the differences between each layer. Remember to **Pause** between each layer.

After you have cleared the seven heart layers with the 1st Chakra move your hand up to the 2nd and then the 3rd Chakra repeating the clearing as above.

Heart Layers and the 4th Chakra

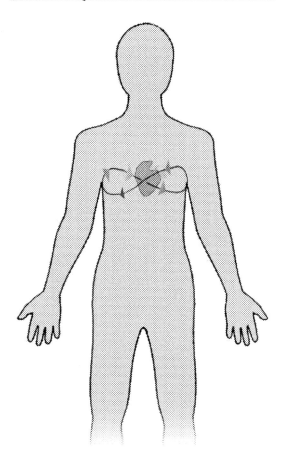

<u>When we clear the heart layers with the 4th Chakra the procedure changes.</u>

Instead of connecting the heart layers with the 4th chakra using a vertical Flowing 8 we will be using a <u>horizontal</u> Flowing 8.

This change in direction helps us clear the Yin and Yang aspects of the 4th chakra in a very powerful way.

Heart Layers and the 5th, 6th and 7th Chakras

After you complete clearing the 4th chakra using the <u>horizontal</u> Flowing 8, return to the <u>vertical</u> Flowing 8 to clear the heart layers with the 5th, 6th and 7th chakras.

Chapter Review

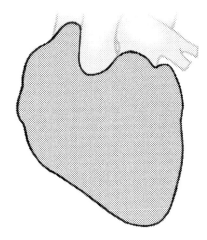

Our Heart

Is the center of our circulatory system.

Is a major endocrine gland.

Starts beating within 20 days after conception even before our brain has been formed.

Can act independently of the cranial brain and has extensive sensory capacities.

Generates an extremely strong, intense signal which is stronger than any other signal produced by any other part of the body.

Sends more information to the brain than the brain sends to the heart.

The electromagnetic center of the body with an electromagnetic field (EMF) that is five thousand times stronger than that of the brain.

Has an electrical field that is sixty times greater than that of our brain.

Is the first line of communication. Incoming information first impacts the heart, then goes through the heart, to the brain and then the rest of the body.

Is the center of our body, as well as the home of our soul.

<u>Heart Quotes</u>

"The best and most beautiful things in the world cannot be seen or even touched – they must be felt with the heart."

Helen Keller

"There is no exercise better for the heart than reaching down and lifting people up."

John A. Holmes

"As the wisest of sages have always realized, the root of essential being is in the heart."

Michael Latorra

"The place to improve the world is first in one's own heart and head and hands and then work outward from there."

Robert M. Pirsig

"Words are just words and without heart they have no meaning."

Chinese Proverb

"It is only with the heart that one can see rightly; what is essential is invisible to the eye."

Antoine de Saint-Exupery

"A loving heart is the truest wisdom."

Charles Dickens

Chapter 8

Life Lines

"One should be always on the trail
of one's own deepest nature.

For it is the fearless living out of your own
essential nature
that connects you to the divine."

Henry David Thoreau

Introduction

We are all beings of light.

Put another way, we are spiritual beings having a human experience. As children, most of us know this. But as we get older, we have forgotten what and who we really are and cannot remember our true nature.

Instead, we are taught that our true nature is not real and are encouraged to forget our truth.

As a result, we are lead to believe that magic is not real, that our invisible playmates do not really exist, and that we are limited beings with only one earthly life to live.

There is enormous pressure to conform to this concept of ourselves, and so we lose touch with our full potential, forgetting that we are powerful beings of light.

From the moment of conception, when our soul's essence joins the energy from our parents, this life's journey begins.

Our energetic life line flows from time in the womb to birth, through early childhood, childhood, teenage years and into adulthood.

Anywhere along our lifeline that traumatic events transpire (as experienced from that age view point), disharmonies may be created that slow down our vibrational flow within.

Also remember that when the clarity of our essence merges with the heavier vibration of the earth's energy, it can be quite a jolt to us.

Our goal is to clear away these distortions throughout the entire life line, so that the power of our essence can flow freely to the present and be used for our highest good.

Let's begin our journey!

Our Life Line

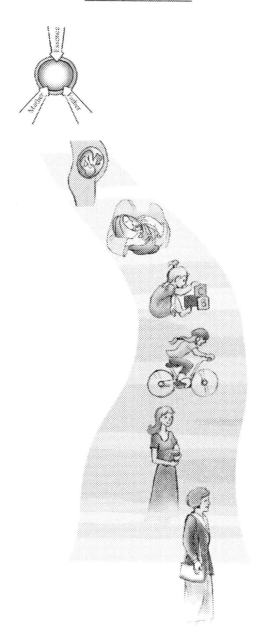

Our Life Line takes us from conception to the present moment.

On the following pages we will review each of the major areas of our journeys. Please take time to review your journey. You may wish to record your journey on separate pages so you can expand where needed and save them for future review.

Conception

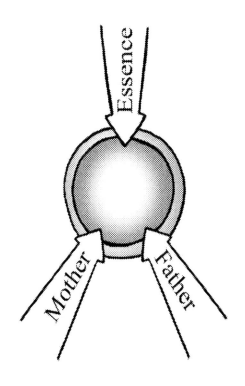

At the time of conception, we are imprinted with the vibrational energies of our own essence and the energetic blueprints of our mothers and fathers.

These blueprints are the vibrational memories that have gone unresolved in both of our parents' journeys. These memories are recorded throughout our bodies.

So as we begin our physical journey, we can see that the vibrancy of our Essence is distorted (masked) by our parents' history.

Take a few minutes and think back to any remembered issues that your parents may have experienced, and shared, from weeks before and at the time of your conception.

Examples:

Was this pregnancy planned and or wanted?

Financial crisis or wars?

Death or loss of loved ones?

Separation from family?

What events happened in your family?

_____

_____

_____

_____

Womb

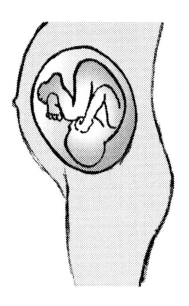

As you began your development within your mother's womb, your heart began to record the events that surrounded your parents (as early as 20 days after conception).

During this time, the un-harmonic events that happened to them also happened to you, even though you have no conscious memory of the events.

Examples:

Financial hardships

Separation of loved ones due to work or wars

Death of love ones

Local or national tragedies

Extended family events

Was your mother on medications that created disharmony?

What events happened during your mother's pregnancy with you?

Exercise

Conception and Womb

Before beginning, and at the end of a session, be sure to ground your client.

To clear the distortions held in these portions of the Life Line, we will connect to the client's umbilicus. This connection can bring up lots of emotions just by placing your hand there. Therefore, be very gentle with your approach and touch.

Allow the energy to align with you while holding the connection with the umbilicus for a few moments before you begin.

Conception

While holding the umbilicus, set your intention to clear any distortions held at conception. First focus on your client's essence and clear *.

> Did this focus bring up any old issues that still need to be released?

Next focus on their mother and clear *.

> Did this focus bring up any out of balance vibrations?

Now focus on their Father and clear *.

> Did this focus bring up any out of balance vibrations?

*Use your thoughts (or your free hand) to move the energy using the Full Body Energy Flow. Repeat the FBEF until any distortions are clear.

Womb

While still holding the umbilicus, shift your focus to clear issues held from time in the womb *.

*Use your thoughts (or your free hand) to move the energy using the Full Body Energy Flow. Repeat the FBEF until any distortions are clear.

If there seem to be multiple issues held from the Womb time, break down the time by clearing each month.

Note: In some clients, these times can be traumatic due to many outside events. It may take several sessions to fully clear these events. Do the best you can at a session, and know that each layer you clear helps that person have more vibrancy in their life.

Birth

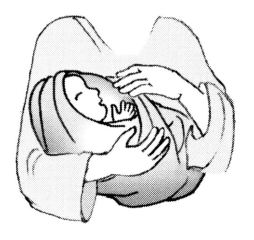

Most families remember the birth of their children as a happy event.

But in reality, physical birth is a major trauma to the mother and the new baby.

The numerous disharmonies that may occur are recorded by your body and heart.

Examples:

Was your mother awake or sedated?

Was your birth your mother's first, and associated with unknown fears?

Was labor long?

Was labor induced?

Was excess force used to assist delivery?

Was the environment of the birthing facility calm or chaotic?

Do you know of any events that happened during your birth?

_____

_____

_____

_____

_____

Early Childhood

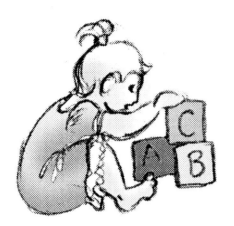

From birth to approximately age six.

During our early childhood development, our conscious mind - or our rational thinking mind - is **not** engaged while it is in the process of being developed.

Events that take place during this time are recorded in our subconscious (our bodies) as real truths because our mind is unable to filter the good from the not so good.

Because of this and the environments (i.e., family, towns, parts of the world) we grow up in, we believe many things about ourselves that are really not factual.

Examples:

Boys are better than girls

Children are to be seen and not heard

You are not as pretty or as smart as others

Your brothers or sisters are better than you

How long before your mother returned to work?

Were you breast or bottle fed?

What events do you remember from your early childhood?

_____

_____

_____

_____

_____

Life Lines

Exercise

Birth and Early Childhood

Before beginning, and at the end of a session, be sure to ground your client.

To clear the distortions held in these portions of the Life Line, we will be connecting to the client's umbilicus and the 1st Chakra.

Hold the connection with the umbilicus for a few moments before you begin clearing to allow the energy to align with the connection.

Birth

While holding just the umbilicus, set your intention to clear any distortions held from Birth. First focus on the time leading up to the actual birth *.

Did this time of preparation hold any old issues that still need to be released?

Next focus the time of actual birth *.

Did this time of major trauma leave any vibrations out of balance?

Now focus on the hours after the actual birth (umbilicus and 1st Chakra).

Did this time of new transition leave any vibrations out of balance?

*Use your thoughts (or your free hand) to move energy up from the Earth Chakra using the Full Body Energy Flow to clear any distortions.

Early Childhood

While holding just the 1st Chakra shift your focus to clear issues held from Early Childhood *.

*Use your thoughts (or your free hand) to move energy up from the Earth Chakra using the Full Body Energy Flow to clear any distortions.

If there seems to be multiple issues held from birth to approximately age six, break down the time by clearing each year.

Note: In some clients these times can be traumatic due to many outside events. It may take several sessions to fully clear these events. Do the best you can at a session, and know that each layer you clear helps that person have more vibrancy in their life.

Childhood

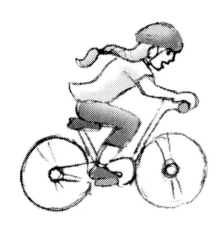

From age six until approximately age twelve.

During our childhood years, our conscious mind or rational thinking begins to engage. This process allows us to begin looking at, or weighing, the events and information that happen around us.

We begin desiring to make our own decisions and choose who and what will be part of our life.

Also at this time, we are required by family, teachers and friends to fit into certain standards of actions, dress and who to associate with. This can be challenging because we want to belong while still wanting to decide for ourselves.

Examples:

Join a team because a friend or parent plays

Select friends because someone we know says they are the ones to know

Wear certain styles because they are in

Do something we know we shouldn't just to be liked

Act out to be noticed

What events do you remember from your childhood?

_____

_____

_____

_____

Teenage Years

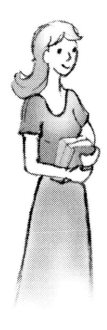

From approximately age 12 until approximately age 21.

During the development of our teen years, conscious and rational thinking has developed to the point of being able to evaluate truths from falsehoods.

At this time, the body is affected by enormous hormonal influences. These influences distract the conscious mind from the evaluation of truths or falsehoods. This hormonal period is also the start of the transition from dependent childhood to independent adulthood.

Even though we can see a truth, we may wish to experience a non-truth to show our individuality. Though this time seems like rebellion, it is actually a time of self-discovery. Hopefully, most events during this time do not leave lasting imbalances.

Examples:

Over conformity to peer pressure

Extreme rebellious activities

Over indulgence of alcohol, drugs, or tobacco

Intimacy experimentation

High or low expectations from family

Was your family stable, or were you required to take on adult duties?

What events happened in your teenage years?

_____

_____

_____

_____

Exercise

Childhood and Teen Years

Before beginning, and at the end of a session, be sure to ground your client.

To clear the distortions held in these portions of the Life Line, we will connect to the clients' 2nd and 3rd Chakras.

Hold the connection with the Chakras for a few moments before you begin clearing to allow the energy to align with the connection.

Childhood

While holding the 2nd and 3rd Chakras, set your intention to clear any distortions held from Childhood (age six until approximately age twelve) *.

*Use your thoughts (or free hand) to move energy up from the Earth Chakra using the Full Body Energy Flow to clear any distortions.

If there seems to be multiple issues during Childhood, break down the time by clearing each year.

Teen Years

While holding just the 3st Chakra, shift your focus to clear issues held from the Teen Years (age 12 until 21) *.

*Use your thoughts (or free hand) to move energy up from the Earth Chakra using the Full Body Energy Flow to clear any distortions.

If there seems to be multiple issues during the Teen Years, break down the time by clearing each year.

Note: In some clients, these times can be traumatic due to many outside events. It may take several sessions to fully clear these events. Do the best you can at each session, and allow the clearing to release some of the accumulated issues and lighten the remaining congestion for the next session.

Life's Potential

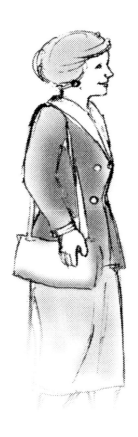

Now that you have made it through your birth, childhood and teenage years you now begin your conscious journey.

We head out to achieve the dreams that we wish for and make a positive place in the world.

But as you have seen in the time leading up to this juncture, many events have taken place which have created subconscious programs that can hold you   back from your true potential.

As we begin to have conscious experiences, some of them bring more imbalances to our vibration because they respond or attach to existing distortions already recorded in our bodies.

What have been some of the major events in your adult life that have created distortions to your harmony?

Physical Events: (Injuries, surgeries, major accidents, war, births)

_____

_____

_____

_____

_____

Life's Potential continued

Mental Events: (Relationships, work, health, money, children)

_____
_____
_____
_____
_____

Emotional Events: (Relationships, work, health, money, loss of loved ones)

_____
_____
_____
_____
_____

Spiritual Events: (Loss of loved ones, unfulfilled life, lack of direction)

_____
_____
_____
_____

Take your time to list as many events as you can remember. This review not only helps you to be aware of imbalances you may be carrying, but also how events have contributed to the imbalances that your clients may be carrying.

Hopefully, this exercise will also give you patience with your own healing too!

Life's Potential Exercise

To clear the distortions held in this portion of the Life Line, we will connect to the client's heart. While holding the heart, set your intention to clear any distortions held from the Life's Potential or Adult Years.

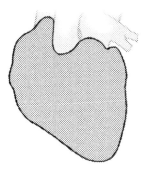

Use your thoughts (or your free hand) to move energy up from the Earth Chakra using the Full Body Energy Flow to clear any distortions in 10 year increments.

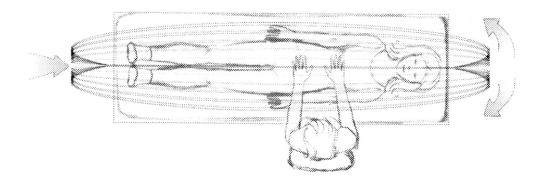

If there seem to be multiple issues during any portion of the Life's Potential, break down the clearing into five year or even single year increments.

At the end of the session be sure to ground your client.

Chapter Review

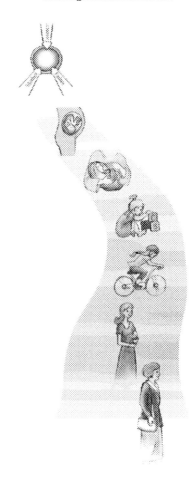

Our energetic Life Line takes us from conception to the present moment.

I hope each of you has taken, or will take, time to write down the major events that have occurred in your own journey.

By taking the time to review your own journey, it helps you see areas of your journey where additional healing can be directed to increase the flow of your essence into your everyday life.

By writing down your own journey, you will also become more aware of various events that can take place very early in a person's journey. These early events may still be directing your actions even though you have no memory of them. This awareness can be very helpful when working with present or future clients.

Appendix

"Praise bright blue skies

and dark rain clouds.

Lift happy voices

upon the morning air.

Murmur sweet words softly

in the evening breeze.

Be present in all things

and thankful for all things."

Maya Angelou

Suggested Reading List

Cellular Memory

Bruce H. Lipton, Ph.D., The Biology of Belief
  Unleashing the Power of Consciousness, Matter & Miracles

Candace Pert, Ph.D., Your Body is Your Subconscious Mind

Babette Rothschild, The Body Remembers
  The Psychophysiology of Trauma and Trauma Treatment

Joan C. King, Ph.D., Cellular Wisdom
  Decoding the Body's Secret Language

Energy

Donna Eden, Energy Medicine (specifically ISBN 1-58542-021-2)

Lynne McTaggart, The Field
  The Quest for the Secret Force of the Universe

Cyndi Dale, The Subtle Body
  An Encyclopedia of Your Energetic Anatomy

Chakras

Liz Simpson, The Book of Chakra Healing

Caroline Myss, Ph.D., Anatomy of the Spirit
  The Seven Stages of Power and Healing

Gateways

Takeo Takahashi, Atlas of the Human Body

Heart

Doc Childre and Howard Martin, The Heartmath Solution

Misc.

Masaru Emoto, Hidden Messages in Water
Louise L. Hay, You Can Heal Your Life
20th Century Fox DVD, What the Bleep!?
  Down the Rabbit Hole – One Movie, Infinite Possibilities
CD recommendations are included in Self Care on page 18

A Journey to Healing

For all the Ladies

The Dangers of Underwire Bras

by Megan Intfen

August 22, 2013

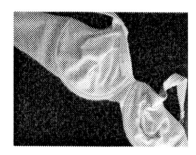

You've heard the risks of wearing an underwire bra, right? Aside from the fact that they are uncomfortable, difficult to find the right fit, and come with the constant threat of puncturing your poor breasts, underwire bras are a serious health concern. There's a lot of research out there dispelling this claim, alleging that there have not been enough studies (read *Western Medicine* studies) that support throwing out your wires. However, I'm inclined to believe holistic women's health pioneers Dr. Joseph Mercola, Dr. Christiane Northrup and my mentor and Energy Medicine guru, Donna Eden. They, like most Eastern Medicine practitioners, find that not only do underwire impede the drainage of lymph, but they also inhibit the flow of *qi*, which is, you know, only your basic life force energy.

Bras in general, especially those worn too tightly, inhibit the movement of lymph. Since lymph is the major highway of toxins, and toxins from antiperspirants and other beauty products tend to hang out around the breasts, you really want your lymph flowing smoothly and easily. Below each breast is a series of neurolymphatic points associated with the Stomach and Liver. Toxins and energy tend to accumulate in these points, causing them to be painful. Over time, cysts can develop in these areas, which are often a precursor to breast cancer.

Go ahead, give a little rub under your breast and see if these points are sore. If so, keep rubbing and drink plenty of water to chase those toxins out.

For all the Ladies Continued

Metal is the other issue with underwire bras. Having a hard metal wire pressed against your neurolymphatic points for long periods of time over-stimulates those points, eventually sedating the organs associated with the points and pulling electromagnetic energy to the area.

Toxins, cysts, over-stimulated neurolymphatic points, and excessive electromagnetic energy ...no wonder women who wear underwire are much more likely to get breast cancer! For their book *Dressed to Kill: The Link Between Breast Cancer and Bras*, Sydney Singer and Soma Grismaijer' conducted a study on women who wear bras versus those who don't. The findings are shocking. Women who don't wear bras at all were nearly *125 times* less likely to get breast cancer than those who always wear them. Yikes!

While going totally braless is not an option for us heavily-endowed ladies, you CAN wear bras that will cut your risk significantly. First, make sure your bra is not too tight. It shouldn't leave red marks under your boobs or cut into your skin. Second, go wireless. Buy wireless bras or cut the wires out of the ones you own. Lastly, take the damn thing off when you get home and let the girls' breath!

Take it from me, a former lingerie designer and undergarment snob, there are plenty of good brassieres out there that don't contain a death wire and are still capable of holding up your boobs. Wacoal, Warner, Vanity Fair, Sassybax and even good ol' Vic's Secret have wireless options. My favorite choice for anyone D cup or under is Gap Body. They have a whole line of inexpensive wire-free bras.

There's no cure for cancer, my sisters, so let's focus on prevention. Protect your girls!

My thanks to Megan Intfen, www.energyhealingnyc.net, for allowing me to include her great article in my handbook.

Training Program Overview

Description

The *Clearing Held Memories* Training Program presents a unique form of energetic bodywork. This work is a complimentary and integrative energy therapy program.

Goal

Participants will develop and strengthen their understanding and application of the *Clearing Held Memories* principles, techniques and energy systems.

Courses

Laying the Foundation   40 CE Hours

Participants will learn how to apply six energy movement techniques to multi aspects of five primary energy systems.

Class 1 – Energy Flow & Chakras
Class 2 – Expanding Energy Flows
Class 3 – Gateway to Emotions
Class 4 – Energies of the Heart
Class 5 – Life Lines

Pathways of Emotions   40 CE Hours

Participants will learn how to apply energy movement techniques to the Gateway connections located along the Pathways.

Class 1 – Energetic Meridians
Class 2 – Emotional Pathway I
Class 3 – Emotional Pathway II
Class 4 – Emotional Pathway III
Class 5 – Flowing with the Pathways

Mastering Vibrations   40 CE Hours

Participants will acquire advance procedures to master assessing and applying energy techniques.

Class 1 – Advance Pathways
Class 2 – Elements of Emotion
Class 3 – Spinal Energy
Class 4 – Advanced Life Lines
Class 5 – Fields and Layers

Practitioner Levels

Practitioner I

Participants must complete all classes of "Laying the Foundation" and "Pathways of Emotions".

Practitioner II

Participants must complete "Mastering Vibrations" and receive the Instructor's recommendation.

Certified Practitioner

Participants must be a Practitioner II.
In addition they must provide documentation of a minimum 50 CHM sessions, obtain a minimum of 10 hours of mentorship and receive recommendation for certification from an instructor.

Instructor

Certified Practitioners may become an Instructor of the Clearing Held Memories Training Program. Applicants must student teach with a certified Instructor and be approved by the Director of Training.

Training Program Endorsements

I am writing to enthusiastically endorse Bruce Winkle and his training program *Clearing Held Memories*. I have known Bruce as a patient for several years, and over this time I have come to appreciate the depth of his clinical knowledge and incredible compassion for others. His work reflects a true enthusiasm for helping others heal, and provides an educational structure regarding energy work that is thorough and thoughtful.

I have had many years of training and involvement in energy-based modalities, first as a Five Element Shiatsu practitioner, and subsequently conducting clinical trials examining Qi Gong and Reiki at the University of Michigan. Bruce is clearly an expert in this area, and I feel has the ability to contribute significantly to the field.

> Andrew Heyman, MD MHSA
> Adjunct Assistant Professor
> Program Director of Integrative and Metabolic Medicine
> The George Washington University
>
> Virginia Center for Health and Wellness
> Aldie, VA

I am pleased to endorse Bruce Winkle and his *Clearing Held Memories* training program.

I have known Bruce as a friend and a patient for about ten years, and have always found him very good in the field of energy work and training healers. In addition, Bruce has a great compassion for the healing arts and combines it with his excellent clinical experience that are reflected well in his program. I strongly believe that Bruce is a good instructor and his program is well prepared.

> Tuan Anh Nguyen, Ph.D., L.Ac.
>
> ACUPUNCTURE & HERB CLINIC, LLC.
> Sterling, VA

Training Program

NCBTMB Approved Provider

The *Clearing Held Memories* Training Program is approved for Continuing Education by the National Certification Board for Therapeutic Massage and Bodywork (NCBTMB).

The program contains three 40 CE Hour courses that provide you with the knowledge and techniques of this unique form of energetic bodywork. This program is a complimentary and integrative energy therapy program.

In Person Participation

Classes are offered in a classroom setting for in person attendance. Each class is taught in a one eight hour day with lots of hands on practice.

Testimonial

I'm always looking to improve and add to my skills as a holistic practitioner.

I'd heard about cellular clearing and I wanted to explore its potential as a therapeutic modality. As a certified reflexologist, adding this protocol to my holistic methods only enhances the benefit my clientele experience.

I can provide deeper layers of stress and emotional release because of the application of the techniques learned in the *Clearing Held Memories* training program.

Jilliana Raymond – New Bern, NC
Certified Reflexologist, Teacher, Author,
CHM - Practitioner II, NCBTMB approved provider.

Distance Learning

The *Clearing Held Memories* Training Program classes are also available via **live, interactive,** internet webinars. These classes are presented in two – four hour units which allows participants from multiple time zones to join in.

Testimonial

I want to say that the online webinar class was absolutely fantastic. I loved the flexibility of the course as it allowed me to still be at home for my work and family.

Traveling across the nation for coursework can be a significant cost, and being able to save this money and not worry about hotels, car rentals and plane tickets allows me to budget for more education.

The interactive webinar itself was outstanding! Bruce is a phenomenal instructor and being able to have that face to face conversation while learning the techniques is just like being in a small setting class in person. I was able to see what he was doing and hear him clearly, and with high speed internet on both ends, the conversation is seamless.

I love Bruce's approach to energy work as he recognizes that each individual is different and incorporates different ways to see, learn and experience his techniques. I felt that his approach was founded over a very broad and diverse education and brought together a better understanding of energy work and how that can tie into our bodies from the past into the "now." Whether you are new to energy work or are looking for more depth to the energy work you already do, this is a great course.

As a massage therapist, this has added another layer to my bodywork and my clients have been over the moon with how connected they feel and how much less "force" is needed to "dig" out what has normally been "tough, chronic issues."

I will be back to attend more coursework, it is worth every bit.

Deborah Jaouen - Glenwood Springs, CO
LMT, CPMS, Doula

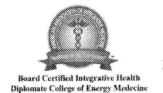
Bruce Winkle
Energy Healer, Teacher and Author

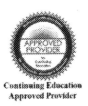
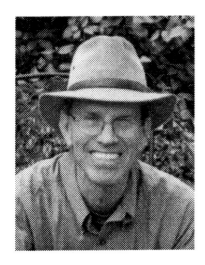

I became an energy practitioner in 1997 and have worked extensively with both people and animals. I feel my work with horses greatly expanded my connection and understanding of energy.

In 1999, I became a Reiki Teacher, and began teaching all levels including Level I & II at NOVA in Sterling, Virginia.

In 2001 I began creating a series of energy medicine courses including: Advanced Energy Medicine, Energetic Wellness for Horses and Clearing Held Memories.

In 2004, I introduced Reiki to the oncology department at Inova Loudoun Hospital in Lansdowne, Virginia and continue to coordinate the practitioners at the monthly Reiki Cancer Support group. In addition it has been my privilege to work in nursing homes and with hospice patients.

I have attended a wide variety of healing workshops and seminars to build my understanding and knowledge of energy medicine including:

> Anatomy and Physiology with Sue Hovland RN, BSN, CMT
> Biology of Cells with Dr. Bruce Lipton
> Energy Healing with Dr. Adam "Dream Healer"
> Energetic Healing with Dr. Mary Jo Trapp Bulbrook (Levels 1 – 7)
> Healing Touch with Maureen McCracken (Level 1 - 5)
> Reiki - Levels I, II, Master and Teacher
> The Reconnection Healing – Levels 1 and 2 with Dr. Eric Pearl
> Knowledge exchange with an acupuncturist trained in China

I continue to study diverse energy modalities so I can continue to bring the best to my clients, students and readers.

Please visit my web site, **www.brucewinkle.com** , for ongoing classes, other events and additional information.

You may email me at **bruce@brucewinkle.com** or call me at 703-771-7755 if I can assist you in your journey.